*S*HAPING UP

DURING AND AFTER PREGNANCY

DR STAVIA BLUNT MA, MRCP, PhD

Copyright © Dr. Stavia Blunt 1997

Summersdale Publishers
46 West Street
Chichester
West Sussex
PO19 1RP
United Kingdom

A CIP catalogue record for this book is available from the British Library.

ISBN 1 84024 013 X

Printed and bound in Great Britain by Wessex Press Group, Ltd.

*To my mother, Elly, who started my interest
in so many things in life, including the
pleasure of physical activity through yoga;
and to my husband George and children
Peter and Elly - because of whom the material
in this book came about!*

ACKNOWLEDGMENTS

Melissa Brake
Penny Burgess-Smith
Fiona Burnett
Rebecca Profit

PHOTOGRAPHS

Richard Wise
Keith McClelland LMPA

COVER DESIGN

Java Jive Design,
Chichester.

CONTENTS

FURTHER INFORMATION

FOREWORD

The modern woman can look forward to pregnancy with the confidence that she will cope with the natural changes that the birth experience will bring her. She will be supported by a society of friends and family and by caring professionals skilled in her needs at this special time. There will still be many anxieties and among these will be the desire to maintain good physical health during the pregnancy. Diet and exercise which are always important will be especially so during this time. A strong wish to return to pre-pregnancy looks and not to put on extra pounds is often a major point of conversation. Most mothers want to get 'back in shape' as soon as possible after the birth of their baby.

Much advice is available and often freely given, sometimes influenced by fashion and fad. This book offers common sense advice about diet and exercise based on personal experience and sound medical facts. It will appeal mostly to the woman who wishes to make her own contribution to the success of her pregnancy and to her future health and appearance.

This book will also be a useful reference for those of us who give advice to the pregnant mother and to answer some of the many questions today's mothers are asking.

It gives me great pleasure to recommend Dr. Stavia Blunt's book which makes such an important contribution to maternity health. Please read it. It will be time well spent.

Anthony D. Haeri, FRCS, FRCOG
Consultant Obstetrician
Ealing Hospital NHS Trust.

Honorary Consultant
Imperial College, Hammersmith Hospital.

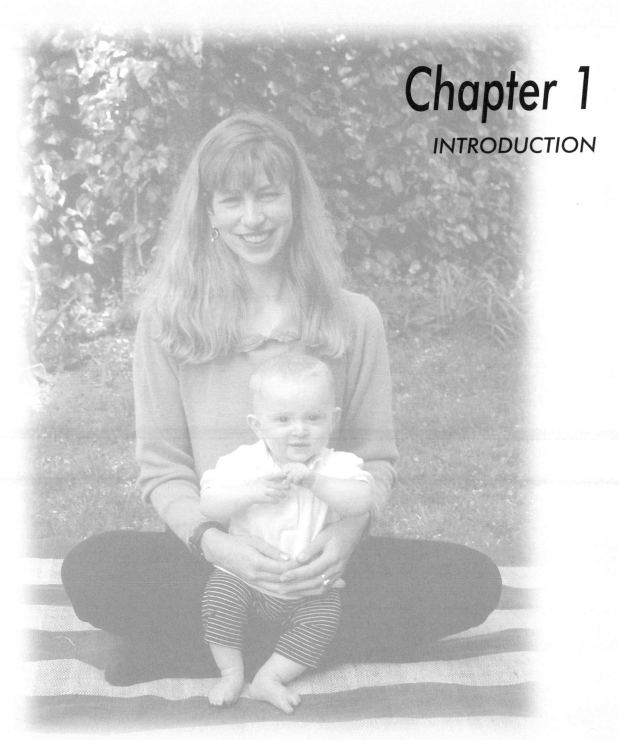

Chapter 1

INTRODUCTION

Pregnancy and childbirth can be wonderful experiences, but, inevitably, reproduction results in extensive changes to our bodies and also to our approach to life. The health of the mother both before and during pregnancy is crucial to the outcome of the pregnancy for the mother and for the baby. So, the healthy way to begin a pregnancy is when the mother is well nourished, eating a balanced diet and is physically fit and active. A healthy lifestyle and absence of excessive stress are also important.

Pregnancy does require that the mother gains a minimum amount of weight in order for the baby to grow and develop adequately. Many women fear that pregnancy will make them flabby, stretched and overweight, and this can be a strong disincentive for getting pregnant in the first place! Many studies have shown that unless women return to their pre-pregnancy weight and physical condition within the first 6 months of delivery, they are unlikely to do so after that. In other words, any excess weight at 6 months may be permanent.

You should, I hope, be prepared and in a position to prevent permanent weight gain from occurring and I am sure that you are looking forward to getting your body back in shape. This book will help make that possible. The information provided on diet, weight change and physical activity is medically accurate. The exercises were developed by me during my maternity leave, after the birth of my second child, and they use my knowledge of anatomy and the physical and hormonal changes that occur during and after pregnancy.

These exercises have really worked for me. With the correct approach before, during and after pregnancy, there is no reason why you should not return to (or even improve upon!) your pre-pregnancy shape and state of health.

What the book covers

- The major hormonal and physical changes that happen during pregnancy, after delivery and during breast feeding.

- Nutritional advice for the mother during and after pregnancy.

- The ideal body weight and how to achieve it.

- Physical activity during and after pregnancy.

- Health, diet, and physical appearance after pregnancy.

- And, of course, the exercises to get you back in shape!

Diet and exercise are two of the most important factors which will influence your return to your pre-pregnancy condition. Whilst you can modify the diet at home (provided you have sufficient information) a regular amount of physical exercise can be difficult to organise, particularly if it involves a class when arrangements for looking after the new baby will need to be made.

It is far less painful to expose oneself to the critical eye of the mirror in the privacy of your own home and so, for this reason, all the exercises in this book can be done at home. The aqua exercises could be tackled once you have got your figure and confidence back!

The exercises

The exercises are arranged in three stages with the levels of physical demand gradually increasing. There are exercises for immediately after birth, for the first 6 weeks after delivery and then for 6 weeks and onwards. These last exercises are designed to 'finely tune' your shape. There is a special section for those mothers who have had a caesarean section.

The exercises

- Are *not* strenuous and are *not* designed to improve aerobic capacity.

- Are aimed at maintaining mobility and suppleness.

- Will help improve your muscle tone and strength, as well as helping you achieve relaxation and so relieve stress.

- Will help with common problems of backache and poor posture.

- Are designed with the physical changes that occur during pregnancy in mind.

It is probably a good idea to try and read the book through a couple of times before you start on the exercise programmes so you can familiarise yourself with the movements.

You will soon be back to looking your best, if not better. The exercises in this book will give you great self-confidence and also give you the energy and strength that you need to cope with all the demands of the new baby!

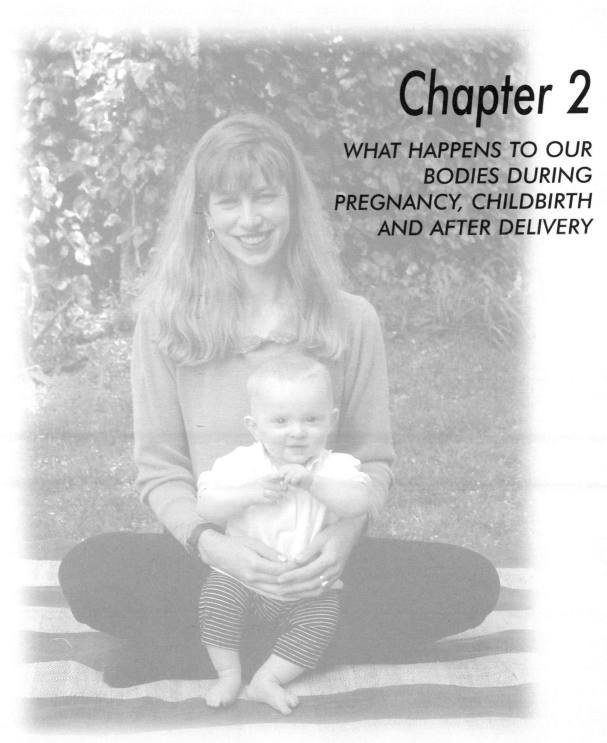

Chapter 2

WHAT HAPPENS TO OUR BODIES DURING PREGNANCY, CHILDBIRTH AND AFTER DELIVERY

This chapter summarises the changes that take place to our bodies during pregnancy, childbirth and breast feeding. For more information see the appendices at the back. The information in this chapter is not a substitute for a detailed text on pregnancy, but focuses solely on those aspects which are of particular relevance to the physical changes occurring in the mother.

During pregnancy, a number of important changes take place. The implantation of the fertilised egg in the uterus begins a series of hormonal changes which cause drastic modifications to the metabolism of the mother. These hormones cause physical changes in the mother's body which are designed to provide the optimal environment for the baby.

In any normal pregnancy there will be

- An increase in size of the reproductive organs (uterus and breasts).

- An increased blood volume and tendency to retain fluid.

- An increased work load for the heart and kidneys.

- Alterations in the breathing pattern, appetite and eating habits, and also mood.

- There is increased fat distribution as part of the overall weight gain.

- Enlargement of the abdomen causing stretching of muscles and skin.

- Postural changes.

HORMONAL CHANGES

The menstrual cycle is controlled by a number of hormones (chemicals released into the blood eg by the ovaries or the pituitary gland in the brain, and which travel to another part of the body where they have a particular effect).

In pregnancy, some of the 'female' hormones of the menstrual cycle increase in amount, whilst other pregnancy-specific hormones begin to be produced. These female 'sex' hormones and the pregnancy-specific hormones are produced by the ovaries and later in pregnancy, by the placenta.

Since these hormonal changes are largely responsible for the changes that occur to the mother's body during reproduction, the functions of some of the most relevant hormones will be summarised below.

Changes also occur to other hormones which are not specifically 'female', but which have a general effect on the way in which cells work, and the metabolism of the body. Some of these are relevant to the major physical changes in the mother, and the effects they produce will also be explained.

Oestrogens

Oestrogens exist in different forms in the body. In the non-pregnant state, they are produced by the ovaries. In pregnancy, the production of oestrogens is mainly by the placenta.

Oestrogens have many important functions in both the pregnant and non-pregnant woman:

- Oestrogens stimulate the formation of protein (essential to growth and maintenance of body tissues).

- They increase our tendency to retain fluid.

- They are responsible for certain sexual features (i.e. breasts, uterus, vagina).

- In pregnancy, oestrogens stimulate the growth of the uterus.

- They increase the size and mobility of the nipple.

- They stimulate egg production in the ovary and the development of the gland (milk-producing) tissue in the breast.

- At the onset of labour, oestrogens stimulate the uterus to contract.

Oestrogen levels increase markedly during pregnancy. After delivery there is a dramatic fall in levels of oestrogen, with resulting major 'involutional' changes in the uterus (i.e. a gradual shrinking back towards the pre-pregnant size), and in the metabolism of the mother. In addition, this fall in oestrogen after delivery may contribute to the depression that is a common feature in the post-natal period.

Progesterone

Progesterone is another hormone that is normally produced by the ovaries during the menstrual cycle, but which is mainly produced by the placenta during pregnancy. Small amounts are also produced by the adrenal glands.

Progesterones also have many important functions in both the pregnant and non-pregnant woman:

- Progesterone stimulates development of the lining of the uterus and causes a thickening of the 'mucous' (ie. the watery secretion) that is produced by the cervix.

- It causes the smooth muscle (a particular type of muscle in the body that the uterus, stomach, bowels, bladder and the walls of blood vessels are made from) to relax. The relaxing effects of progesterone on these muscles explains many of the features seen during pregnancy: veins on the surface of the skin and in the breasts become more prominent, and constipation is common. This effect on blood vessels is one reason why the blood pressure may fall when progesterone levels are high (such as during the second half of the menstrual cycle, and in pregnancy) and why women tend to faint more easily during those times.

- Progesterone also stimulates the development of the glandular tissue in the breasts.

- It causes a rise in body temperature (a finding that is often used in diagnosing pregnancy) and increases respiration.

- The hormone is also thought to have a 'calming' effect during pregnancy.

- It also has an effect on the mother's immune system preventing her from 'rejecting' the fetus.

Progesterone levels increase markedly during pregnancy. After delivery of the baby, as with oestrogen, the level of progesterone in the mother's blood falls, and so the effects on the mother's body are reduced.

Human chorionic gonadotrophin

HCG is involved in stimulating steroid hormone metabolism, and also contributes to the development of the breasts. It may be responsible for the nausea that is common in early pregnancy. Levels of HCG in the mother's blood fall after delivery to pre-pregnancy levels.

Human placental lactogen

The main role of HPL is to divert more of the glucose in the mother's blood towards the developing baby. HPL is also involved in development of the glandular tissue of the breasts, and may be involved in triggering the onset of milk production. After delivery, with the loss of the placenta, levels of HPL fall again to pre-pregnancy levels.

Oxytocin

Oxytocin is a hormone produced by the pituitary gland in the brain during pregnancy and breast feeding. It stimulates the onset of labour by its action on the uterus. A synthetic form of this hormone ('syntocinon') is often used for induction of labour. Oxytocin's main role after delivery is in ejecting milk from the breasts during suckling (the so-called 'let-down' reflex).

Prolactin

Prolactin is another hormone produced by the pituitary gland. Its main role is during breast feeding when it stimulates the growth of breast tissue and maintains milk secretion.

Other hormones

A number of other hormones alter during pregnancy. These changes affect the mother's metabolism and ensure that appropriate modifications are made to the mother's own use of nutrients in her diet.

During pregnancy, all these hormonal changes contribute to many of the specific features of pregnancy such as:

- Softened and enlarged uterus
- Prominent distended veins
- Enlarged tender breasts
- Increased size of the areola
- Increased size and mobility of the nipple
- Urinary frequency
- Vomiting and nausea
- Weight gain
- Mood changes
- Increased metabolism and appetite

Hormonal Changes After Delivery

After delivery, dramatic changes occur because of the loss of the placenta, which has been producing most of the above hormones during pregnancy. The ovary does not begin to take over hormone production immediately after delivery. Thus, levels of oestrogen, progesterone, HCG and HPL fall massively, as does the tendency to retain fluid. Levels of other hormones, such as prolactin and oxytocin, remain high or increase, because of their role in breast feeding.

These hormonal changes contribute to the rapid early weight loss that occurs after delivery, and are followed by a progressive 'involution' of the uterus, whereby it gradually shrinks back towards its pre-pregnant size. Similar involutional changes also occur in the vagina, which becomes less 'swollen'. The fall in hormone levels after delivery, especially oestrogen, contribute to the mood changes that are common after delivery. Changes in hormone levels after delivery stimulate milk production which begins on about day 3 after delivery. For more detailed information on hormonal changes during and after pregnancy see *Appendix I*.

CHANGES TO THE BODY DURING AND AFTER PREGNANCY

The uterus, cervix and vagina

- During pregnancy the uterus increases in weight from about 65g to about 1Kg at the end of the nine months. The increase in size is not only due to growth of the uterus wall and lining, but also due to distension by the growing baby and amniotic fluid.

- The blood supply of the uterus also increases.

- The cervix increases in size, softness and blood supply.

- The vagina, vulva and perineum (the area between the vagina and anus) become softer and relaxed, and more swollen due to an increase in blood supply. This increased blood supply to the perineum can sometimes result in varicose veins of the vulva and vagina in the same way that 'piles' can occur around the back passage during pregnancy.

   During the three months after delivery, the uterus gradually shrinks back towards its pre-pregnant size ('involution'). Breast feeding increases the speed at which this involution occurs. The cervix and vagina also gradually revert back to their pre-pregnant size.

Breasts

- Pregnancy hormones cause a thickening of the skin of the nipple, enlargement of the pink areola, and growth of the underlying gland tissue.

- There is an increased blood supply and deposition of fat in the breasts especially around the glandular tissue.

- The nipple enlarges and becomes more erect.

- The areola and nipple may darken especially in dark skinned women. This pigmentation may persist after pregnancy.

- Stretching of the skin of the breasts may produce stretch marks and drooping of the breasts. The extent to which breasts increase in size during pregnancy varies enormously. Some women notice a change in bra size.

- The breasts tend to become tender especially during the early weeks of pregnancy.

After delivery, as milk production is being established, the breasts enlarge still further and can become very uncomfortable. The size fluctuates with the frequency of breast feeding and in relation to the previous feed. Once breast feeding has ceased completely, the breasts usually shrink in size, but the final size reached is variable. Breasts may return to their non-pregnant size, or they may remain larger, but in some cases they end up being smaller than they were before pregnancy.

Breast sagging following pregnancy and breast feeding is a common complaint. The best way of minimising this is by trying to prevent further stretching of the skin beyond that which occurs as a result of the increased size of the breasts. Breasts sagging under their own weight will aggravate stretching.

Wear a strong supportive bra with thick firm straps throughout pregnancy and breast feeding, and possibly also at night.

Fat deposition

Weight gain during pregnancy results from a combination of the products of the pregnancy (ie the enlarged uterus, the baby and the amniotic fluid), increased fluid and blood volume, and increased fat.

Unfortunately, for most women this is more easily said than done, especially when most mothers are more concerned about providing adequate nutrition for their baby during pregnancy than they are about their figure! Many women gain more weight during pregnancy than they should, and this excess weight is harder to lose afterwards. (This topic is discussed in more detail in Chapter 3.)

During pregnancy, fat tends to be deposited in the typical 'prone areas' - over the breasts, hips, bottom, upper thighs and upper arms. Some of these fat stores are important in supplementing the energy content of breast milk in breast feeding mothers, and are therefore valuable. However, once the baby's needs are no longer of concern, there is no further need for the mother's excess fat stores to stay. Appropriate diet and exercises specifically designed for these areas are effective ways of removing any excess fat deposition in the months after delivery.

Abdominal wall

During pregnancy, the abdomen increases progressively in size due to the growing uterus, baby and amniotic fluid. This results in gradual stretching of the abdominal wall and, within the abdomen, the normal contents (such as the loops of bowel, the bladder and the liver) are pushed aside by the growing pregnancy. The contents of the abdomen seem to cope remarkably well with this!

As the abdomen grows, the skin over it becomes stretched, and sometimes stretch marks can appear. A pigmented line known as the linea nigra, running between the belly button and the top of the pubic bone, also often appears; this may persist after pregnancy in some women. Recent advertisements advocating the use of 'anti-stretch mark creams' have no valid scientific basis, although their use may help to keep the skin supple, and they are soothing. Some of these creams contain 'antioxidants' such as vitamins A and E, which may have a role in preventing some of the ageing changes in skin.

In addition to stretching of the skin, other parts of the abdominal wall are stretched during pregnancy. The abdominal wall is made up of skin, a layer of fat, and then a complex series of muscles, which are shown in figure 1 opposite.

The muscles run in 3 main directions (the **rectus muscles** - vertically up and down the front of the abdomen; the **transversus muscles** - across the abdomen; and the **internal and external oblique muscles** - diagonally). The activity of these muscles is important because they act like a 'biological corset' keeping the contents of the abdomen firmly in place, and also maintaining the waist line. The other main function of the abdominal muscles, together with many smaller muscles that run along the length of the spine (the paraspinal muscles), is to maintain a firm, erect posture.

Diagrams of the Abdominal Wall Before and After Pregnancy

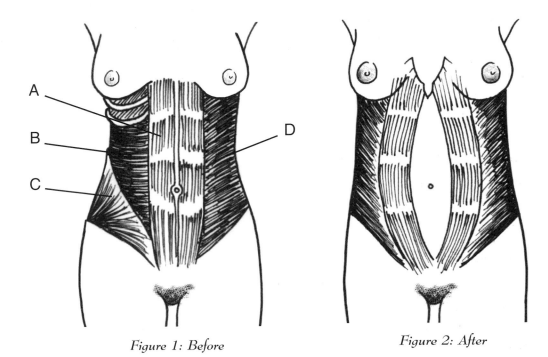

A

B

C

D

Figure 1: Before

Figure 2: After

Key to the muscles

A: Rectus abdominis	C: Internal oblique
B: Transversus	D: External oblique

As the abdominal muscles become stretched during pregnancy, the rectus muscles split down the middle along a fibrous sheath (the linea alba) which normally bridges the two parts of the rectus muscles together. After delivery, a gap is still usually present (figure 2, above).

Using the exercises in this book will help tighten the abdominal muscles. It is possible for the rectus muscles to return to the pre-pregnant condition and for the gap to close completely, and measurement of this gap is a useful guide as to how effective your exercises are. The improvement in muscle tone can also be measured by keeping a check on waist width and circumference.

The resulting gap that develops cannot be felt so easily during pregnancy, but it is readily felt afterwards. You can feel it by lying on your back, and raising your head and upper body gently off the floor (figure 3, below).

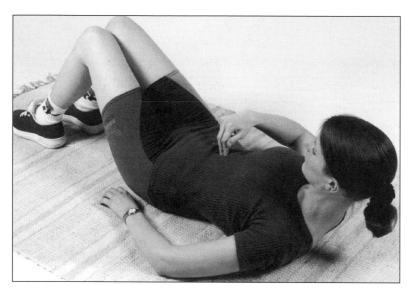

Checking the gap between the two bands of rectus muscle - after delivery this gap may be several finger breadths wide. With gradual strengthening and toning of the abdominal muscles, the rectus muscles should gradually come together and the gap should close.

This makes the two rectus muscles tighten, and if you place your finger tips just above the belly button, you may feel a gap of about 3 fingerbreadths shortly after delivery.

Damage to the abdominal wall as a result of caesarean section

The degree of damage to some extent depends on whether the operation is done as an elective (i.e. planned procedure) or as an emergency. Most planned and emergency caesarean sections are performed through a relatively small lower abdominal incision, but occasionally larger incisions are required. Such incisions involve cutting through the entire thickness of the abdomen as well as the wall of the uterus. Stitches are inserted after the operation, but complete healing of the wound can take 2 weeks or longer. During this time the mother will feel uncomfortable and will need a lot of assistance. The extra damage to the abdominal muscles means that more demanding exercises have to be delayed (usually by at least 2 weeks) compared with women who have had a vaginal delivery.

Spine, posture and pelvic joints

Good posture depends on the interaction of the bones and ligaments of the spine, the muscles running the length of the spinal column (which enable the spine to bend, and also to keep it erect), and the muscles in the neck and abdominal wall.

> **Good posture is important because it**
> - Minimises the strain put on the bones and joints of the spine.
> - Reduces the chances of developing back pain.
> - Reduces the chance of developing osteoarthritis in later life.
> - Looks good.

Good posture does not happen on its own. It requires conscious effort at first, until it becomes second nature. Pregnancy is bad for posture for a number of reasons. As the baby grows and the breasts enlarge, our centre of gravity is pulled forwards, and we tend to lean backwards to compensate.

The changes to the spine during pregnancy are shown in figure 4 (right).

The result is that the spine is pulled forwards at certain points, which exaggerates its normal curvature . These changes can result in backache, and muscle imbalance and spasm along the spine.

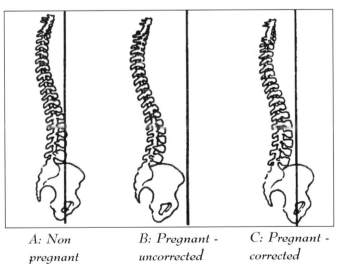

A: Non pregnant

B: Pregnant - uncorrected posture

C: Pregnant - corrected posture

Poor posture often continues after pregnancy as some women may be afraid to 'stand tall', especially if there have been perineal stitches or a caesarean section. This fear is unfounded. The exercises in this book are aimed specifically at retoning and tightening these muscles to help you achieve excellent posture and a wonderful figure.

Figure 5a and 5b, below and opposite: Diagrams of the pelvic floor muscles and ligaments in relation to the openings of the bladder, vagina and back passage.

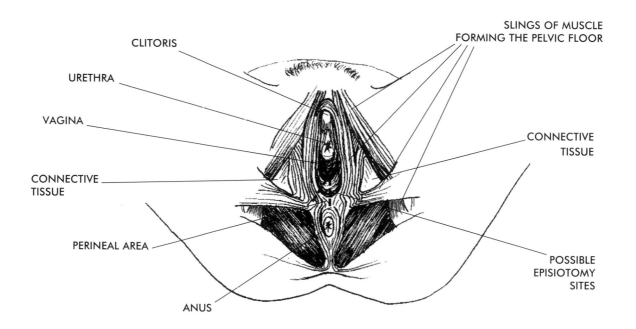

CLITORIS

URETHRA

VAGINA

CONNECTIVE TISSUE

PERINEAL AREA

ANUS

SLINGS OF MUSCLE FORMING THE PELVIC FLOOR

CONNECTIVE TISSUE

POSSIBLE EPISIOTOMY SITES

Stretching and damage to the pelvic floor and perineum

The pelvic wall is made up of the pelvic bones, muscles and skin. The muscles which form the floor of the pelvis are very important because they help to support the contents of the pelvis (the uterus, vagina and bladder). The pelvic floor muscles are also important in control of the front and back passages. Ligaments stretching from the walls of the pelvic cavity also strengthen the pelvic floor, and these become softer during pregnancy. The muscle and skin that form the perineal area and entrance to the vagina are also important in enjoyment of sexual intercourse.

The muscles of the pelvic floor originate from the pelvic bones (which form the 'sides' of the pelvic cavity) and meet in the middle, making a sort of 'sling' of muscles between the opening out of which urine comes (the urethra), the vagina and the anus (figure 5a).

Good tone in these muscles is important. Mild weakness of these muscles can result in vague aches and pains or feelings of heaviness

Figure 5b, below: Side view.

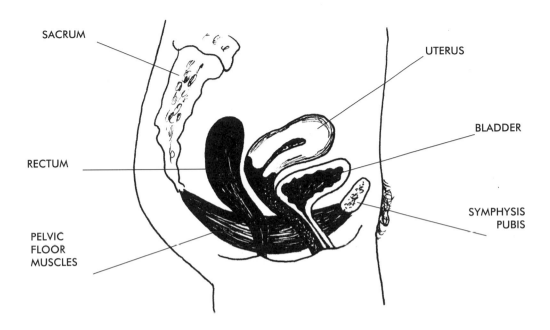

SACRUM

UTERUS

BLADDER

RECTUM

PELVIC
FLOOR
MUSCLES

SYMPHYSIS
PUBIS

(all of which are aggravated during pregnancy when there is excess fluid and blood supply to the area). More severe weakness can result in collapse of the bladder and inner walls of the vagina.

In addition to the muscles forming the pelvic floor, the small openings from the front and back passage, out of which urine and faeces pass respectively, are surrounded by two very important rings of muscle, known as 'sphincters'. The activity of these sphincters allows us to have careful, fine control over when we open our bowels and when we urinate. These sphincters, and the remaining muscles forming the pelvic floor are under our voluntary control (i.e. we can make them contract and relax when we want to), and the correct functioning of the sphincters is essential for preventing incontinence.

The skin of the perineum, and the muscles of the pelvic floor and the sphincters can become stretched, torn or cut during pregnancy and childbirth respectively.

Older women, and those who have had multiple vaginal births are more likely to have serious problems such as incontinence and uterine prolapse following damage to the pelvic floor. A poorly repaired perineum can also cause discomfort and problems with sexual intercourse after pregnancy. Chapter 6 describes exercises which can help to prevent stretching of the pelvic floor muscles, and which re-tone damaged muscles and help to heal the perineum.

Eating habits

Both during and after pregnancy bad eating habits often develop. Food intake during pregnancy and whilst breast feeding often far exceeds requirements as the mother feels that she has to eat for two! We will look at diet and weight in the next chapter. Furthermore, urges to eat certain foods can be troublesome. Sometimes the presence of nausea alters eating habits because some women find that the only way of relieving it is by eating.

Mood

During pregnancy, hormones work in such a way that many women become more relaxed mentally, more 'placid' and often simply feel more content. After delivery, mood changes can occur and depression can sometimes interfere with the mother's determination to return to her pre-pregnant state. This can then result in a vicious circle. If you are feeling depressed for prolonged periods or to any moderate degree, then seek assistance.

Tiredness

Pregnancy can be tiring because of the increased energy demands placed on the mother. Pregnancy hormones also increase the tendency to feel sleepy, whilst, on the other hand, sleeping (especially in the later weeks of pregnancy) can be difficult and easily disrupted because of the size of the abdomen. Some women also become tired because of nutritional insufficiency.

After delivery, the reasons for tiredness are different: labour itself is physically exhausting and constant attention is needed for the new baby; sleep may be interrupted, and sometimes nutritional deficiencies may develop. The sudden changes in hormone levels may also contribute.

> **The best ways of overcoming tiredness are to make sure that you are eating a healthy, balanced diet, resting whenever possible, and remember to ask for help!**

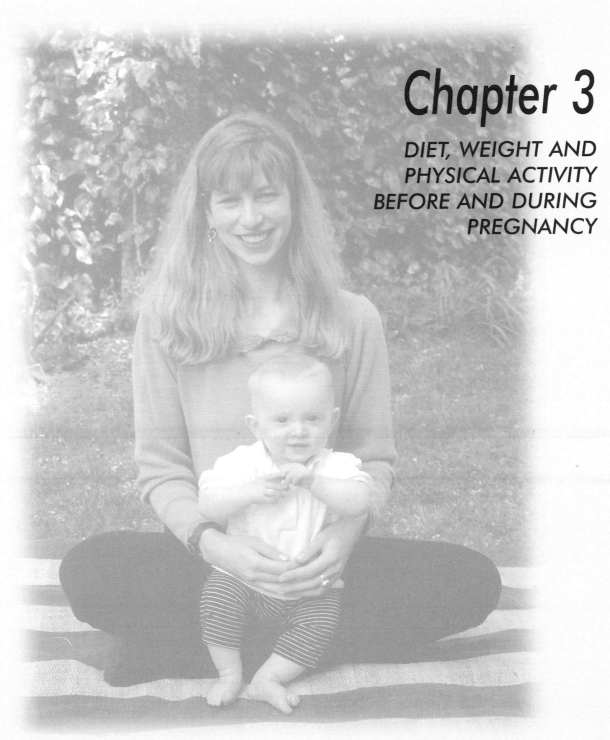

Chapter 3

DIET, WEIGHT AND PHYSICAL ACTIVITY BEFORE AND DURING PREGNANCY

Diet, weight and physical activity are major preoccupations for many women. However, you may well be worried that dieting or excessive exercise during pregnancy and breast feeding may be disadvantageous to your baby. Extremes in weight, diet or physical activity can be harmful to both mother and developing baby, so sound scientific information is required regarding the benefits and risks during the reproductive period.

In this and the following chapter, these three important areas are covered both in relation to pregnancy and afterwards. There is also additional information in *Appendices II* and *III*.

PRE-PREGNANCY

The course and outcome of pregnancy (i.e. the health of mother and baby) are affected by a number of conditions relating to the mother's pre-pregnancy state, such as her general health, lifestyle, weight and height. The best way to begin a pregnancy is when you are in good physical health, pursuing a healthy lifestyle, eating a well balanced diet, and not under excessive stress. Throughout pregnancy, diet, weight gain, lifestyle and physical activity have additional effects on the outcome of pregnancy. Adverse conditions may have adverse effects on the duration of the pregnancy and the birthweight of the baby.

Pre-pregnancy nutrition and diet

A normal balanced diet should contain adequate amounts of protein, carbohydrate, essential fats, vitamins, minerals and trace elements. Provided a normal balanced diet has been followed for some months before pregnancy, adequate body stores of many of these nutrients will have accumulated, without the need for supplementation. If, however, the daily diet is unbalanced, or if the mother is in poor general health, or suffers from a medical condition which might affect food absorption, this will result in excessive loss of these elements and deficiencies in certain nutrients may occur.

Relative deficiencies of certain nutrients occur more readily in women who smoke (eg the requirement for vitamin C is increased), and who drink excessively (requirements for certain B-group vitamins are increased). In the weeks and months leading up to conception, particular attention should be paid to the intake of adequate amounts of iron, folic acid, and vitamin D as the requirements for these nutrients increases tremendously during pregnancy, and it is relatively easy to become deficient in them if the diet has been inadequate before pregnancy.

RECOMMENDED DAILY INTAKE OF IMPORTANT NUTRIENTS BEFORE PREGNANCY

The data in this table is derived from the Food and Nutrition Board (1980), and applies to women aged between 18-50. Provided a well balanced diet is taken, the vitamins and minerals mentioned here will be obtained in sufficient amount without the need to take supplements.

NUTRIENT	MODERATELY ACTIVE WOMEN
Energy (Kcal)	2,150
Protein	44-46g
Calcium	500-800mg
Iron	18mg
Magnesium	300mg
Zinc	15mg
Phosphorus	1200mg
Iodine	150µg
Vitamin A	750µg
Vitamin D	5-10µg
Vitamin E	8mg
Vitamin C	50mg
Folic acid	200-400µg
Niacin	13mg
Thiamin	1.1mg
Riboflavin	1.3mg

Food sources of these nutrients are shown on the following pages.

Pre-pregnancy body weight

The ability to reproduce effectively and healthily depends on the mother's physical growth and development. The onset of periods and the continuation of normal menstrual cycle (and thus fertility) depends on the attainment and maintenance of a minimum weight for height ratio, which reflects a minimum essential store of body fat. Thus, being too thin or obese is not conducive to normal reproductive capacity.

WEIGHT-FOR-HEIGHT VALUES

| Height (in) | Weight (lb) ⟶ | | | |
	Underweight	Normal	Overweight	Obese
57	101	102-133	134-150	151
58	103	104-136	137-153	154
59	106	107-140	141-157	158
60	107	108-142	143-159	160
61	110	111-145	146-164	165
62	113	114-149	150-168	169
63	115	116-152	153-172	173
64	118	119-156	157-176	177
65	121	122-160	161-180	181
66	123	124-163	164-184	185
67	126	127-167	168-188	189
68	129	130-170	171-192	193
69	132	133-174	175-196	197
70	134	135-178	179-200	201

[Handwritten annotations in margin: 12-11-98, 154 lbs (no more than 3 Lbs more), 5'7", and a star mark next to row 67]

Based on the midpoint of the medium frame ideal weight-for-height of the 1983 Metropolitan Life Height and Weight Tables. Statistical Bulletin of the Metropolitan Life Insurance Company, 1983:64:2-9.

Weight-to-height ratio in the non-pregnant state is a good indicator of your weight status (i.e. whether you are of normal, under, or over weight), and these values can be used to predict how much weight should be gained during pregnancy. The table opposite shows the reference weight-for-height values for a medium framed woman, in the pre-pregnant state. This table is useful for identifying where you fall, and for predicting how much weight you should ideally gain during pregnancy.

Pre-pregnancy physical activity

A distinction should be made between physical activity of everyday life (referred to hereon as 'routine activity'), and specific exercises, which are designed to be undertaken in addition to the activities of daily living. The level of routine activity varies greatly between different people, and according to their lifestyles. Some women have very active lives, and are always on the move; others spend much of the day sedentary; and there are those who fall in between. For those who lead sedentary lives, building up a regular exercise routine is one way of ensuring an adequate level of fitness.

Exercise regimes can also vary greatly. Some variables include the physical ease of the exercises, the level of cardiovascular fitness required, the amount of impact or weight-bearing involved, and the amount of strain they exert on bones and joints. Being physically fit prior to pregnancy has obvious advantages because it prepares the mother for the extra energy demands that pregnancy will place on her. Most studies of the benefits and risks of 'exercise' (as opposed to general physical activity as part of daily life) have focused on aerobic exercise, rather than on weight resistance training.

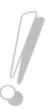

Good general advice

Exercise in moderation, which does not cause pain, discomfort, repeated strain, excessive impact, or excessive fatigue is most probably good for you. It is not advisable, however, to begin an arduous regime in a previously unfit state. Physical fitness should be acquired gradually.

DURING PREGNANCY

Nutrition and diet during pregnancy

This section will outline why certain nutrients are important, how much of each is needed in the diet, and from which foods they can be obtained. For more detailed information see *Appendix II* at the end of the book.

Several components of the diet during pregnancy have been specifically shown to affect fetal growth and development. These include:

- Vitamin A
- Folic acid
- Magnesium
- Calcium
- Long-chain fatty acids (such as those found in fish oils)
- Iron

The nutrients that are at greatest risk of being taken in insufficient amounts include:

- Vitamin B6
- Calcium
- Magnesium
- Iron
- Zinc
- Copper

Fortunately, all of these nutrients are present in readily absorbable amounts in meat, poultry, fish and dairy products - all foods that are recommended in additional amounts during pregnancy.

Energy requirements during pregnancy

The amount of energy available from foods is measured in calories. All foods contain calories, the most concentrated form being fat (animal or vegetable), the second being carbohydrate, and the third protein. Energy is obtained most efficiently from carbohydrate which comes in various forms, ranging from simple sugars to more complex starches such as bread and pasta.

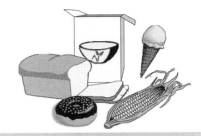

GOOD SOURCES
Sugar, cakes, biscuits, fruits, vegetables, cereals, bread and pasta.

Protein requirements during pregnancy

Proteins are the important 'building blocks' of the body and are especially important during pregnancy and lactation when new tissues are developing.

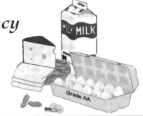

GOOD SOURCES
Meat, fish, eggs, milk, cheese, peanuts, cereals and many vegetables.

Fat requirements during pregnancy

Dietary intake of fat is vital, because fats provide a very concentrated source of energy, and certain types of fat contain essential 'fat-soluble' vitamins (such as vitamins A and D). A minimum of 10% of the diet should be made up of fat to ensure that adequate amounts of these nutrients are absorbed. Fats come in different forms, such as the animal-derived fats, including that found in or next to meat, and in milk products (such as butter); and in fish and vegetable fats including oils and margarine. Fat can also be found as part of a number of foods that are not themselves classified as 'fats', for example lean meat comprises as much as 10% fat.

But, fats are also a highly concentrated form of energy and calories and therefore are potentially very fattening if taken in excess!

FUNCTIONS AND FOOD SOURCES OF VITAMINS

	VITAMIN	FUNCTION	GOOD FOOD SOURCES
A	(retinol or carotene)	Maintains skin and membranes, bones, placenta, vision.	Liver, fish liver oils, whole milk, carrots, dark green vegetables, eggs.
B1	(thiamin)	The B-vitamins are considered together because they have parallel functions and also often occur together in the same foods. They affect protein and energy metabolism.	Meat, cereals, liver, milk, green vegetables.
B2	(riboflavin)		
-	(nicotinic acid)		
-	(folic acid)		
B6	(pyridoxine)		
B12	(cyanocobalamin)		
C	(ascorbic acid)	Important for health of gums; improves the availability of iron in the diet; helps metabolism; important defence against 'free-radical' damage.	Most fresh fruit and vegetables; destroyed by cooking.
D	(cholecalciferol)	Needed for the absorption of calcium and therefore is important for bones and teeth. This vitamin can be formed in the skin by the effect of sunlight.	The main food source is fortified milk.
E	(tocopherol)		Vegetable oils, wheat germ, nuts, green leafy vegetables.

Vitamin requirements during pregnancy

Vitamins are essential to the normal functioning of the body, affecting the ways in which cells work. They are also essential for the normal development and growth of the fetus. There are thirteen known vitamins, and whilst all are essential to life, eight are of special importance because it is relatively easy to become deficient in them as a result of poor diet.

RECOMMENDED DIETARY ALLOWANCE OF VITAMINS

Vitamin		Before/After Pregnancy	During Pregnancy
A	(retinol or carotene)	less than 800µg retinol equivalents Excess intake of vitamin A can be harmful to the fetus, so supplements should not be taken during pregnancy. It is also advisable to avoid foods such as liver, which may contain very large amounts of this vitamin.	
B1	(thiamin)	1.1mg	1.5mg
B2	(riboflavin)	1.3mg	1.6mg
-	(nicotinic acid)	13-15mg	17mg
-	(folic acid)	200-400µg	400-800µg
		The requirement of folic acid more than doubles during pregnancy. High intake before conception may help to reduce the chances of certain fetal malformations. Higher doses should not be taken.	
B6	(pyridoxine)	1.6mg	2.2mg
B12	(cyanocobalamin)	2.0µg	2.2µg
C	(ascorbic acid)	50mg	70mg
D	(cholecalciferol)	5µg	10µg
E	(tocopherol)	8mg	10mg (excessive amounts are potentially harmful)
F	(menaphthone)	65µg	65µg

Adapted from the Food and Nutrition Board, National Academy of Sciences.

- The requirements for folic acid and vitamin D increase by 100% over non-pregnant levels.

- With certain vitamins, in particular vitamins A and D, care should be taken not to consume excessive amounts, as they are potentially harmful to the fetus.

- Vitamin supplements are rarely required during pregnancy provided a normal balanced diet is followed.

Minerals and trace elements requirements during pregnancy

More detailed information is in *Appendix III* at the back of the book.

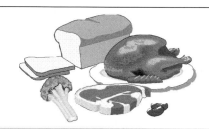

GOOD SOURCES
Red meat, liver, dark turkey, breads and cereals, dried beans and peas, dried figs and prunes, broccoli and spinach.

IRON

Iron is important because it helps red blood cells carry oxygen in the blood, and if there is too little iron, symptoms of anaemia can develop, such as tiredness. Iron also helps the function of many enzymes in the body. Lack of iron can affect not only the mother, but also the growth and well-being of the fetus.

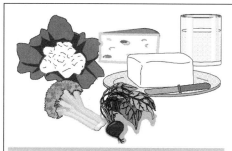

GOOD SOURCES
Dairy products and leafy vegetables.

CALCIUM

Calcium is vital for the development and maintenance of the skeleton, for nerve cell and muscle function, for blood clotting and for the function of most cells in the body. Calcium accumulates with pregnancy, mostly in the baby's skeleton, and especially during the last 3 months of pregnancy. The amount of calcium in the blood depends on the amount of vitamin D available.

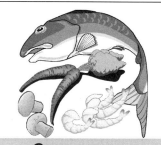

GOOD SOURCES
Sea food, vegetables and some forms of salt.

IODINE

Iodine is an essential part of the thyroid hormones which are especially important for the normal growth and development of the baby. Severe iodine deficiency during pregnancy can severely affect the baby's development. Milder deficiencies can impair the intellectual and physical development of the baby.

ZINC

Zinc is crucial to the normal functioning of cells, and for the normal development of the baby.

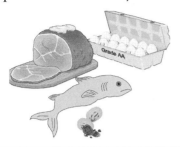

GOOD SOURCES

Animal products such as meat, liver, eggs and some seafoods. Also legumes, seeds, nuts, and whole-grain cereals.

SELENIUM

This is another essential trace element which is important for the function of 'natural antioxidants' (i.e. compounds which 'mop up' harmful products produced in the body).

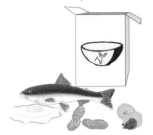

GOOD SOURCES

Brazil nuts, cereals, seafood, offal and eggs.

Fibre requirements during pregnancy

Adequate fibre intake is important at all times of life because it helps to prevent constipation. During pregnancy when there is a tendency to develop constipation, a diet high in fibre can help the problem.

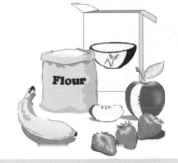

GOOD SOURCES

Most fruit and vegetables, un-refined flours and cereals.

The best way of ensuring an optimal intake of protein, carbohydrate, fat, vitamins and minerals during pregnancy and lactation is the consumption of a well balanced diet that includes both animal and plant food sources. Although vegetarian diets contain reasonable sources of trace elements, flesh foods contain higher levels and in a more readily absorbable form. The same holds true for proteins.

Here, you can see the daily food pattern that should be followed during pregnancy to ensure optimal nutrition.

RECOMMENDED DAILY FOOD INTAKE TO ENSURE OPTIMAL NUTRITION DURING PREGNANCY

Food	*Amount*
Milk, whole	3 x 8oz. glasses
Lean meat, cheese	2 x 4 - 6oz. servings per day
Egg	1
Fruit	At least 2 pieces of citrus fruit or juice equivalent
Vegetables, especially dark green, leafy, and yellow-orange	At least 2 servings per day
Bread and cereals	3 - 4 servings
Vegetable oil, butter, vitamin-fortified margarine	1 tablespoon

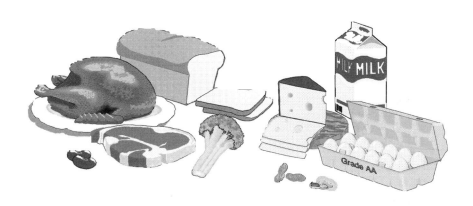

SAMPLE MENU FOR PREGNANCY

Breakfast

1 serving of: Orange juice, cereal or toast, butter or fortified margarine, coffee or tea.

Mid-morning

1 serving of: Orange juice, biscuit, milk (1 or 2 glasses).

Lunch

1 serving of: Meat/cheese with bread or pasta, butter; green vegetables or salad; fresh fruit; milk 4 - 8oz.

Mid-afternoon

Milk (1 or 2 glasses), biscuit or toast.

Supper

1 serving of: Meat or fish with vegetables; single helping of pudding.

Bed-time

Milk (1 or 2 glasses).

Snacks

Raw carrots, fresh fruit, savoury biscuits, cheese.

Diet restriction during pregnancy

Dieting during pregnancy is not advisable even amongst obese women. A low energy intake will impair the growth of the fetus. A lower limit of 15 pounds weight gain (roughly the weight of the tissues comprising the pregnancy) is recommended for obese women, a greater amount for women who are of normal weight before pregnancy, and a greater still weight gain should be achieved by women who are underweight at the start of pregnancy.

Appendix IV covers more details on diet restrictions and weight gain.

Weight gain during pregnancy

During pregnancy, it is normal for the mother's weight to increase. Weight gain during pregnancy, together with the pre-pregnancy weight of the mother, are two of the most important factors determining the weight of the baby at birth. How much weight should be gained will depend on the pre-pregnancy state of the mother.

> **Weight gain during normal pregnancy results from increase in size of maternal tissues such as the uterus, breasts, and body fat, together with the formation of the placenta, amniotic fluid, and the growth of the baby. Fluid retention in the tissues and an increase in the blood volume account for the remaining weight gain. The rate at which growth occurs in these different parts varies with the stage of pregnancy.**

How much weight should be gained?

There is no general recommendation, as the ideal weight gain will vary according to the mother's pre-pregnancy weight. However, there is a clear relationship between the weight of the mother prior to pregnancy, the weight gain during pregnancy, and the birth weight of the baby. Women who are underweight before pregnancy will need to gain more weight, whilst the opposite applies for women who are overweight at the start of pregnancy.

PHYSICAL ACTIVITY DURING PREGNANCY

As with most things in life, extremes of physical activity and exercise are to be avoided. The potential risks and benefits of exercise during pregnancy have been quite extensively reviewed. What has not been examined with quite the same scrutiny, however, is the effect of physical activity that is part of lifestyle or occupation (i.e. what I call here 'routine activity').

Effect during pregnancy of routine activity

Prolonged levels of physical activity such as strenuous effort required in certain jobs are not recommended during pregnancy because they seem to result in a higher incidence of premature labour.

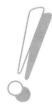

Be careful of	
● Cleaning	● Manual labour
● Carrying heavy loads	● Even prolonged standing

Placental blood flow may suffer during prolonged physical activity, making the potential risk for development of pre-eclampsia and impaired growth of the baby more likely. Strenuous prolonged activity during the last few months appears to be most likely to have adverse effects on the outcome of pregnancy. Moderate amounts of physical activity, to which the mother is already accustomed, are unlikely to have adverse effects on the pregnancy. The general activity resulting from daily living is positively good for the normal pregnant mother, bearing in mind that frequent periods of rest are also required.

A good indicator of how much physical activity is beneficial for any individual is your level of tiredness. Listen to your body - if you feel tired, then you need to rest rather than exercise.

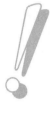

Exercise programmes and pregnancy

Reviews of several studies looking at the effects of exercise programmes on the outcome of pregnancy produced the following advice:

- Any pregnant woman with a medical or surgical condition or obstetric complication should seek medical advice before embarking on an exercise programme during pregnancy. Women who feel chronically tired should not over-exert themselves.

- For women who have undertaken regular exercise prior to pregnancy, it is unlikely that continued exercise during pregnancy will be harmful, unless the exercise is vigorous. However, the risks and benefits of starting a new exercise programme during pregnancy for previously sedentary women are less clear.

- Some women see pregnancy as a time during which their health needs to be optimal, and so, often for the first time, consider beginning a regular exercise regime. This is fine, provided previously inactive women increase exercise frequency and intensity of exercise very gradually.

- Strenuous or prolonged exercise should be totally avoided during the first three months (because abortion can occur) and at other times the duration should not exceed 15 minutes (longer durations can cause temperature rises, reduced blood supply to the fetus, and lower glucose levels in the blood - all of which are harmful for the fetus).

- Exercising in warm and humid temperatures should be avoided.

- Non-weight bearing, and low impact activities (eg cycling on an exercise bike, swimming) should be undertaken in preference to weight-bearing or high impact exercise (eg jogging, combat sports).

- Exercising whilst lying on your back should be avoided after the fourth month of pregnancy.

- Women should drink water before and after exercise to ensure adequate hydration.

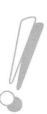

- Exercise should not be undertaken when tired, and frequent rests should be taken to avoid any stress to the fetus.

- How much exercise, and exactly what type of exercise is safe during pregnancy is difficult to establish. Studies have concluded that certain forms of exercise are safe in pregnancy and these have included non-vigorous regimes with aerobics, exercise bike cycling, or swimming for periods ranging from 15-40 minutes 2-3 times per week.

Do you need to exercise during pregnancy?

Some daily physical activity during pregnancy has undoubted benefits, provided it is done in moderation and is in keeping with previous performance levels of the individual. Women who have a moderately active lifestyle (i.e. routine activity) may not need to undertake a specific exercise routine during pregnancy.

> **Any exercise routine that is undertaken in women who are not used to exercise prior to pregnancy should be increased gradually. I do not believe that strenuous or prolonged exercise can be good for pregnancy. Excessive and vigorous exertion can reduce the blood supply to the uterus (because the blood is being diverted towards the mother's exercising muscles instead), as well as the oxygen and glucose content, and so prevent nourishment of the fetus. It can also have harmful effects on the mother's spine.**
>
> **EXERCISES MUST BE UNDERTAKEN WITH CAUTION DURING PREGNANCY.**

For these reasons, the exercises for during pregnancy in Chapter 6 of this book are not exercise programmes in the typical sense. The exercises are aimed more at correcting posture, establishing pelvic floor exercises, breathing, maintaining mobility, strength, and muscle relaxation.

Ensuring adequate rest during pregnancy

It is important to recognise that, whilst physical activity has undoubted benefits during pregnancy, adequate rest is equally important. Blood flow to the uterus and placenta increases markedly when the mother is resting, so increasing the availability of nutrients to the fetus. This means that the pregnant woman should make sure she gets more physical and emotional relaxation per day than she had previously.

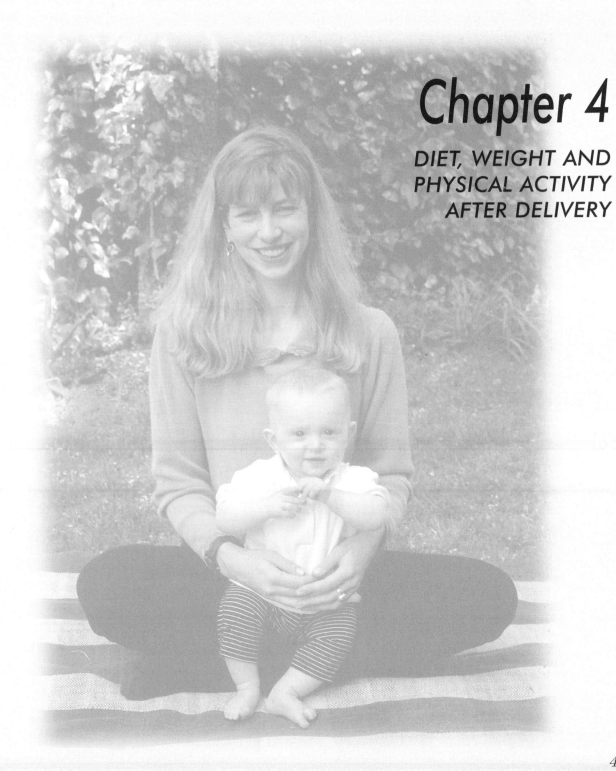

Chapter 4

DIET, WEIGHT AND PHYSICAL ACTIVITY AFTER DELIVERY

P reoccupation with weight and physical appearance is probably at its greatest after birth. This is also one of the most difficult times for you to find the will power and self-discipline to do what it may take in order to lose weight and regain your pre-pregnancy shape. You have a new baby to care for, and you are probably chronically tired. I hope that the advice and information given in this chapter will help you achieve your goals.

Summary of advice and information in this chapter

- Diet during breast feeding

- Weight changes and breast feeding

- Nutrition and diet after delivery

- Balanced energy reduced diets

- Achieving weight loss after delivery

- Effects of physical activity during and after pregnancy

DURING BREAST FEEDING

Diet during breast feeding

Producing milk is nutritionally demanding especially for mothers who breast feed fully for a number of months. The amount of extra food needed by the mother is directly related to the extent to which she is breast feeding. Producing milk uses up about 750 calories per day. The recommendation is that an extra 500 calories per day should be eaten by the breast feeding mother, above those eaten in the pre-pregnant state. The remaining 250 calories is drawn from the accumulated fat stores. Once this store has been depleted, the maternal calorie intake should be increased unless further weight loss is desired.

In addition, the requirements for vitamins A and C, and for iodine and zinc are almost twice those needed during pregnancy. On the other hand, the requirement for folic acid falls back to just above pre-pregnancy amounts. Most of these nutrients are readily available in a well-balanced diet (see Chapter 3) so supplements should not be necessary.

Impact of restriction of maternal diet on breast feeding

This depends to some degree on the mother's nutritional status. Traditionally, it is believed that if the mother's nutritional stores are ample, the exact content of the diet (barring protein) may have little impact on the quality of the milk produced.

However, important nutrients that cannot be stored in the mother's body (such as vitamin C) must be made available daily to the baby via the mother's diet and thus her breast milk.

Content of the diet is thought to have a much more obvious effect on the quantity of milk produced. Reduced fluid intake can also reduce milk production (although too much fluid may have a similarly harmful effect). Breast feeding mothers who wish to produce high quality and quantity milk should ensure a well-balanced diet and should drink adequately.

A safe recommendation for weight reduction is that breast feeding women should consume at least 1800 calories per day. Dieting during the first 2-3 weeks when milk production is being established, and liquid diets at any time, are not recommended.

Weight changes and breast feeding

For those who wish to lose weight whilst breast feeding, providing the mother is well nourished to start with, it seems that attempts to lose weight by moderate physical activity or exercise programmes, and by mild diet reduction are safe and can assist weight loss. What is less clear is whether breast feeding itself has any effect on weight change after birth.

Does breast feeding help weight loss?

In breast feeding mothers, the recommendation that daily intake of calories should increase by 500 calories (rather than 750 which is what breast milk production is thought to require) is based on the rationale that the deficit will be drawn from the mother's excess weight, and so will help her to lose weight. However, some studies suggest that the recommended intake for breast feeding is actually too high, and that milk production does not use up quite as many calories as was thought.

Despite what is commonly believed, the available evidence does not support the notion that breast feeding mothers lose their excess weight faster than non-breast feeding mothers, although this may occur if breast feeding is continued for longer than 6 months.

Does stopping breast feeding help weight loss?

There is practically no information on this important question, although many individual examples suggest that weight loss occurs once breast feeding has stopped.

Physical activity and breast feeding

Much less information is available on the effects of physical activity and exercise regimes on breast feeding than on pregnancy. But, it would seem that moderate physical activity and exercise regimes for a breast feeding mother do not have any adverse effect on the quality or quantity of breast milk, provided an adequate diet is followed.

There is some concern that breast feeding after exercise may be unpalatable for the baby because of higher levels of lactic acid in the breast milk. Most studies suggest that this is only likely to occur after very strenuous and prolonged exercise.

AFTER BREAST FEEDING

Nutrition and diet after delivery and when not breast feeding

Once breast feeding has stopped (or if it never occurred), the concerns that maternal food intake might adversely affect the health of the baby cease. Nevertheless, it is still important that a new mother continues to consume a well balanced diet which contains adequate amounts of all the essential nutrients (see Chapter 3).

Being overweight results from an imbalance between energy intake and energy expenditure. The most effective way of losing weight, therefore, is to eat fewer calories than your body requires, so that fat stores will be used up; and to increase your physical activity (which will burn up more calories). These two elements are the cornerstones of natural, self-directed, weight loss regimes.

DIETING

Provided that nutritional deficiencies have been excluded, and the mother is otherwise in good general health, and can obtain adequate rest, it is probably safe for women after pregnancy who are not breast feeding to follow a diet that would be followed at other times of non-pregnant life. Whatever diet is followed, however, it should be well balanced and nutritionally sound.

What sort of dieting?

There are several different types of diet. They range from fad-diets, fasting, near-starvation, to a high-protein low-carbohydrate diet, to a high-carbohydrate low-protein diet, to a high carbohydrate low-fat diet, to a low calorie balanced diet. Books abound with reports of 'scientific discoveries' that promise to help overweight people shed pounds in a number of days (eg The Cambridge diet, the Macrobiotic diet, the Magic Mayo diet etc).

Crash or fad diets should be avoided because the weight loss is often not permanent and the content of the diet is often nutritionally unsound. Fasting is not recommended because it causes not only loss of fat but also more essential body tissues including muscle, and also a total lack of nutrients is harmful to the general functioning of the body. Drugs should not be used to assist appetite control unless indicated and supervised medically.

The safest and most nutritionally well balanced diet, and the one that I recommend, is a **'balanced energy reduction diet'**. This basically means that the only component of the diet which is reduced is the energy content (i.e. the calories). The number of calories is reduced to the point where the body must draw on its own fat stores in order to meet the body's daily energy needs. The latter will depend on the daily activity of the individual, and will be higher in people who are more physically active.

How does calorie reduction in the diet affect weight ?

As the average woman undergoing normal physical activities uses up between 2000 and 2400 calories per day, and as one pound in body weight is believed to be equivalent to 3,500 calories, it is relatively easy to calculate how much the calorie intake of a diet should be reduced in order to lose a particular amount of weight.

- For a woman of normal activity using up 2000 calories per day (an exercise routine will increase this value), a daily calorie reduction of 500 per day should result in weight loss of one pound per week.

- However, more recent studies have shown that one pound in weight can be lost by an energy deficit of only 2000 calories. Based on this assessment, a dietary reduction of 500 calories per day should cause weight loss of one pound every 4 days, without a change in physical activity.

- Whichever estimate is used, a diet of 1200 calories per day will certainly result in weight loss between 0.5 and 2 pounds per week (depending on activity levels).

How do you know what foods to cut out and what to leave in?

Because the aim is to achieve a diet which is lower in calories but nutritionally well-balanced, and because all foods contain calories, one needs to know which foods one should continue to eat, and which should be reduced or removed from the diet.

For a balanced energy reduced diet

- Fat should be restricted to a minimum

- Carbohydrate to about 150 gm/day

- Protein intake should be high, at about 85gm/day

- Intake of foods containing vitamins and minerals should be high

A sample balanced menu containing approximately 1500 calories, which is high-protein, low fat, and moderate carbohydrate, is shown in the table over the page.

A diet of this nature will certainly result in weight loss over several weeks. Fruit can always be used to replace other forms of carbohydrate, as most fruits and many vegetables have the added advantage that they not only are sources of energy, but they are also high in vitamins.

What diet should be followed for maintaining weight loss?

Obviously, a weight-reducing diet should only be continued for so long as weight loss is required. Once ideal weight has been achieved, the energy intake will need to be increased again in order to prevent further weight loss. On the other hand, once you have lost weight, you will want to keep it off.

SAMPLE WELL BALANCED DIET MENU FOR WEIGHT REDUCTION AFTER DELIVERY AND AFTER BREAST FEEDING HAS STOPPED.

The diet contains 1200 calories of high-protein, low fat, moderate carbohydrate foods.

Breakfast	*Example food*
Fruit	1/2 grapefruit
Bread	2 slices wholemeal
Meat/low fat cheese	1/2 cup cottage cheese
Milk	1 glass semi skimmed
Beverage	Coffee or tea, no milk or sugar

Lunch or supper	*Example food*
Vegetables	2 stalks celery; 1 carrot
Bread	1 slice wholemeal and butter
Meat	6oz lean meat or fish; or a 2 egg omelette
Fruit	1 medium peach
Milk	8oz semi skimmed

Supper or lunch	*Example food*
Meat, lean	6oz grilled meat (or fish)
Vegetable	1 potato; 1/2 cup peas and carrots
Carbohydrate and fat	1 tsp mayonnaise; 1 cup apple sauce
Fruit	1 orange
Drinks	Water, black coffee or tea as desired.

Weight changes after delivery

During pregnancy, most mothers are so concerned that they should be able to supply adequate nutrients to their growing baby, that concerns about their own weight and appearance often take second place. Once concerns about the health of the baby are over, as in after pregnancy, and when not breast feeding, many women are eager to return to their pre-pregnancy weight. One survey showed that as long as 18 months after delivery, 25-40% of women are still on average 9 pounds heavier than their pre-pregnant weight. Loss of excess weight gained after a pregnancy is very unlikely to occur after the first year, so it becomes permanent.

Why excess weight gain is bad for you

It is important to lose the weight gained during pregnancy, and not to gain weight permanently after pregnancy not only because it affects your appearance and self-esteem, but also because carrying excess weight is unhealthy, bringing with it increased risks of heart disease, diabetes, high blood pressure and certain forms of cancer. Excess weight gain also increases the risks in subsequent pregnancies of gestational diabetes, high blood pressure and complications in labour and delivery.

Weight loss in the first 1 to 3 months after delivery

In the first 2 weeks following delivery, women lose on average 10 pounds (roughly the weight of the products of the pregnancy, plus some excess fluid). Following this, the weight loss slows down so that by 4 weeks after delivery, less than one quarter of women have returned to their pre-pregnancy weight. Many women will not have returned to their pre-pregnant weight by the 6 week check.

Weight loss 6 to 12 months after delivery

The weight loss varies hugely during this period between different women, with some returning within a few weeks to their pre-pregnancy levels, others remaining several pounds overweight, and still others who continue to gain weight after delivery.

The biggest risk factor for being overweight after delivery is the amount of weight gained during pregnancy. Excessive weight gain during pregnancy (more than 35 pounds) is very difficult to get rid of.

You are more likely to remain overweight after delivery if you were overweight before pregnancy. Women in their second or greater pregnancy also tend to lose weight more slowly in the first three months after pregnancy. The effect that the age of the mother has is unclear.

How to assist weight loss safely after delivery

PREVENTION
Beginning pregnancy at a normal weight, and gaining the amount of weight recommended for your pre-pregnancy weight are the best ways of ensuring that weight loss occurs after birth.

RETURNING TO WORK
One recent study has shown that mothers who return to work outside the home lose weight more quickly than those who remain at home. The sooner mothers return to work the more rapid is the weight loss.

CIGARETTE SMOKING
Although I would not recommend it under any circumstances, it is a fact that cigarette smoking is protective against excessive weight retention after birth.

SENSIBLE DIETING

SENSIBLE EXERCISE REGIMES

BREAST FEEDING

PHYSICAL ACTIVITY AND EXERCISE

Helping new mothers establish an appropriate exercise routine is an important component of after pregnancy care, and unfortunately may often be neglected. It is well established that mothers who exercise are healthier and leaner than non-exercising mothers, although there is no definite evidence of an enhanced reduction in weight. This may be partly because most of the studies have been done in breast feeding women, who are likely to be on relatively high calorie diets.

Provided there are no medical or obstetric complications, and provided the recommendations shown above are followed, exercises and physical activity, in moderate amounts, after birth, are safe.

Unfortunately, it is often very difficult for a new mother to exercise regularly, especially if she has to arrange child care or expeditions to classes. For these reasons, exercises that can be done in the home provide an obvious solution.

The later chapters in this book provide exercise programmes of increasing demand, appropriate to the different stages. There is a separate section on exercises for women who have had a caesarean section.

ENERGY EXPENDITURE IN CALORIES PER MINUTE BASED ON A 65KG ADULT

Activity	Calories used/minute
Walking slowly	2.9
Walking quickly	5.2
Sitting	1.5
Driving car	2.8
Sweeping floor	1.7
Ironing	4.2
Hoovering	4.8
Cycling slowly	4.5
Cycling fast	11
Active gardening	8.6
Playing tennis	7.1
Swimming	14
Walking in loose snow	20

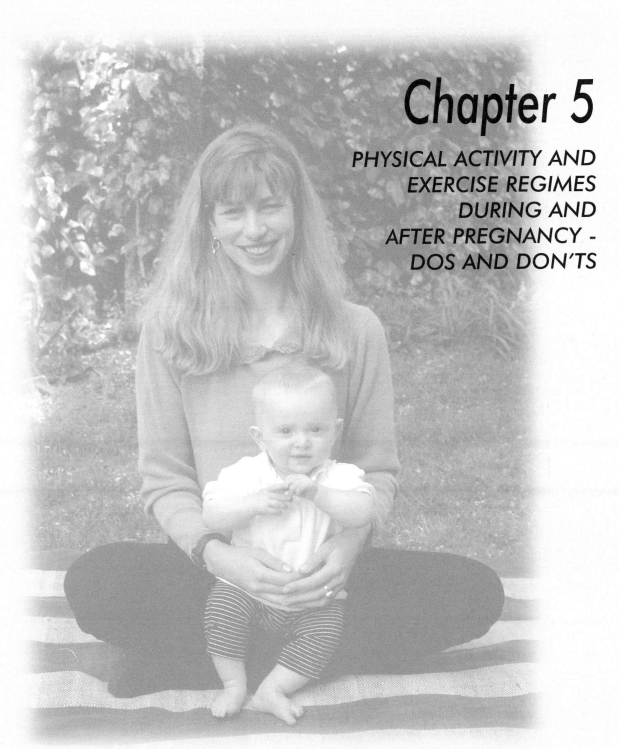

Chapter 5

PHYSICAL ACTIVITY AND EXERCISE REGIMES DURING AND AFTER PREGNANCY - DOS AND DON'TS

PHYSICAL ACTIVITY

Levels of physical activity vary greatly between individuals. During pregnancy, moderate levels of physical activity, provided they are not unusual for that particular individual, are most probably good for you. However, exercise or physical activity should be avoided if you feel tired or unwell. If a change in level of activity is attempted during pregnancy, compared with the pre-pregnant state, then it is most important that this change occurs gradually. The same applies after pregnancy although here it is not so critical because the health of the baby would no longer be at risk.

Excessive physical activity (such as heavy labouring work, jobs involving prolonged standing) are associated with shortened duration of pregnancy, lower birthweight of the baby, and an increased incidence of pregnancy related high blood pressure. It can also have harmful effects on the spine. At all times, therefore, prolonged or strenuous physical activity should be avoided as these can have harmful effects on both the mother and the developing baby.

Summary of advice and information in this chapter

- Exercise programmes during pregnancy
  - What is safe
  - What to avoid
- General guidelines for exercising during pregnancy
- General guidelines for after pregnancy
  - Standing, lifting and moving correctly
  - Exercising
- Learning the exercises

Exercise programmes during pregnancy

During pregnancy, provided levels of physical activity are moderate, it may not be necessary to undertake a specific exercise programme. However, there are specific exercises that are of definite benefit to the pregnant mother, and her ability to cope with labour.

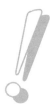

> **In this book, the exercises recommended for pregnancy are not aimed at improving aerobic capacity. They will help tone and strengthen the muscles, improve posture and prevent back ache, aid the control of breathing, muscle relaxation and maintain mobility and the suppleness of muscles and ligaments.**

There are also specific exercises aimed at the pelvic floor and there is a section on aqua exercises. To maintain a general level of fitness, I recommend gentle swimming once or twice a week. Excessive exercise regimes during pregnancy have the same adverse effect on pregnancy outcome that too much physical activity does, and should be avoided.

General guidelines for exercise or physical activity during pregnancy

Exercise or physical activity during pregnancy should not be undertaken if there are any adverse obstetric or medical reasons - if you are uncertain about your fitness to carry out exercise or physical activity check with your doctor.

In moderation, these are believed to be safe during pregnancy

Relaxation	Walking
Muscle toning	Swimming

Avoid any of the following throughout pregnancy

Vigorous aerobics	Bicycling on ordinary terrain
Jogging, skating or riding	Diving
Activity involving high vibration	Contact sports
High impact or high speed activity	

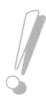

Exercises for the pregnant woman should be:

- In keeping with previous fitness level

- In short spells rather than prolonged bouts

- Avoided in the heat

- Preceded by adequate warm up and warm down

- 'Comfortable' at all times

Any pregnant woman who is suffering from any of the following should not commence any exercise or physical activity regime unless approved by your doctor:

- Heart disease

- Acute infections

- Multiple pregnancy

- Incompetent cervix

- Problems with the growth of the baby (intra-uterine growth retardation)

- High blood pressure

- Bleeding from the vagina/uterus

- Ruptured membranes

- Thyroid disease

- Diabetes

- Previous inactivity

Specific exercises after delivery

It is not essential for a woman to undertake an exercise programme after pregnancy, but such regimes increase the likelihood and speed with which the mother returns to her pre-pregnancy weight and shape after delivery. As mentioned in the previous chapter, however, any exercise programme should be gradual if the mother has not previously been someone who exercised regularly.

> **Any exercise programme which you choose to follow, especially if it is aimed at burning large amounts of calories should be checked for safety according to the guidelines mentioned before.**

The exercises described for after pregnancy in this book are not designed to burn up large amounts of calories, although of course they will help. The exercises continue to work on the same lines as those recommended for during pregnancy, such as posture, pelvic floor strengthening and muscle relaxation techniques.

The post-pregnancy exercises in Chapters 8 and 9 are specifically aimed at toning and strengthening the abdominal muscles, and muscles of the chest wall, the arms, shoulders and leg muscles, and the muscles of the back and spine. The exercises consist of standing and floor exercises, together with a section on dumb-bell exercises which can be done as strength is built up. These exercises will help to tone and shape the body.

Aerobics and high impact exercise do not form any part of the regimes shown in this book. If you want to improve your cardiovascular fitness, I recommend regular swimming which will, together with the exercises described in this book, increase your stamina, suppleness and strength, and will also help to improve your appearance.

If you are breast feeding, it is a good idea to feed your baby just before exercising so that you feel comfortable and your breasts do not leak. The effects of exercise on breast milk production and feeding have been discussed in detail in the previous chapter.

GENERAL ADVICE
Standing and moving correctly

Whatever exercise regime you decide to follow, and even when standing still or carrying out normal activities of daily living, there are correct ways of doing things, and certain things to avoid.

Remember the following tips

When standing:

- Stand as 'tall' as you can, with shoulders back, chin and neck high.

- Tummy and bottom should be tucked in.

- Knees should be relaxed and not forced or 'locked' back.

When lifting follow this sequence:

- First, hold tummy in, back straight and head high; brace the pelvic floor and hold bottom in.

- Next, with back straight, bend knees to a squat, or a kneel.

- Then bring the weight of the object you intend to lift close to your body.

- Finally use the muscles in your legs to lift you slowly back to the standing position.

- Never lift when bending forward, or to the sides.

When moving around generally:

- Avoid sudden twists to the spine and neck.

When exercising

Exercises should be done with proper care and attention so that problems are avoided. Exercises that are incorrectly performed can, in the short term, cause 'pulled muscles', strained ligaments, damaged or ruptured tendons, and even slipped discs. In the longer term, incorrectly performed exercises, or excessive exercise can cause excess wear-and-tear to joints and soft tissues of the body. Of most importance, probably, is the potential effects of incorrectly performed exercises on the spinal cord and the nerve roots. Thus, any movements of the back and neck should be smooth, slow and unforced. Specific guidelines are detailed below about how to perform certain movements and exercises.

Some general advice about exercising

- Do not exercise if you feel tired or unwell.

- Do not exercise if you have a medical or surgical complaint, unless the exercise regime has been approved by your doctor.

- Do not exercise if you have any doubt about your capacity to carry out the exercise safely.

- Do not do 'neck rolls'.

- Do not do 'the windmill'.

- Do sit-ups with knees bent and feet flat on the floor - never with legs straight or feet held down (eg under a bar).

- When doing squats or lunges, always keep the thigh parallel with the floor and try to keep your knee above the ankle; never do deep lunges or deep knee bends (knees should never be bent more than 90 degrees).

- When using weights do controlled slow movements, not fast jolty ones.

- Avoid jerky, bouncy or high impact exercises.

- Avoid sudden twists to the spine or neck.

- Make sure you are well-hydrated before starting.

- Stop if you feel strained or tired.

What You Will Need For The Exercise Regimes

- A comfortable, loose outfit (leggings, T-shirt)

- Bare feet or gym shoes

- An exercise mat, or thick rug or carpet

- A pair of 3 pound dumb bells

- A high backed chair

- Access to a swimming pool for the aqua exercises

If possible, always try and exercise in front of a large mirror.

Learning the Exercises

The exercise routines are arranged as a programme for each stage. Chapter 6 covers the exercises during pregnancy. Chapter 7 covers the exercises for the first 48 hours after delivery, then, when you are ready, the exercise programme in Chapter 8 can be started. Once these exercises have been mastered with ease (this may take around 6 weeks), you can move on to the more demanding programme shown in Chapter 9.

With each exercise there is a detailed description of how to do it, plus an illustration or photograph to help you see exactly what you should be doing. Where relevant, the exact areas and muscles involved in a particular exercise are shown.

Read through the book before you begin. The exercises for pregnancy are to be done in your own time, and any single part can be done on its own. For the exercises after pregnancy, I suggest you try as much as you can working through from beginning to end, and adding more exercises in as you build up your strength.

Do the exercises as many times per week as you can, but don't worry if you are only exercising once a week - it's better than not at all!

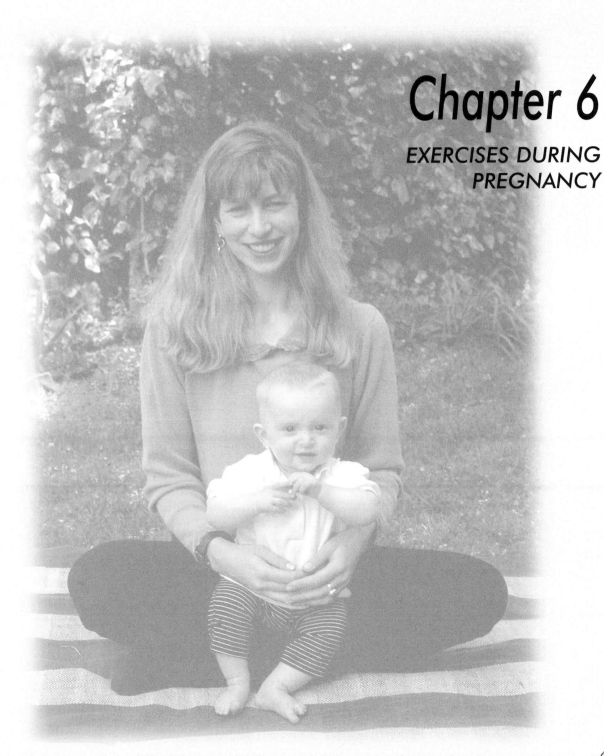

Chapter 6

EXERCISES DURING PREGNANCY

Although these exercises have been put together in a chapter aimed at pregnancy, most of these exercises are also useful after delivery and can be 'dipped into' from time to time as required.

The exercises described here are not part of a programme designed to burn large numbers of calories. They are instead aimed at improving posture, preventing backache, coping with altered muscle tension or muscle imbalance, and improving breathing patterns. Any specific muscles that are used by a particular exercise will be mentioned.

Swimming and aqua exercises can be used to improve cardiovascular fitness and aerobic capacity during exercise, and a simple programme is described here. Exercises for the pelvic floor are also outlined, as it is best to familiarise yourself with what the muscles of this region feel like before they become bruised and sore as a result of childbirth.

During pregnancy,

- I recommend that posture checks be performed every day.

- Exercises for backache and relaxation should be performed as the need arises.

- Pelvic floor exercises should be be done daily.

- The water exercises can be done as often as you like.

POSTURE

Posture describes the way in which you hold your body. In exercise terms it refers to a dynamic position in which the body parts relate to one another in such a way that the centre of gravity is over the base, and the muscle work required to maintain that position is reduced to a minimum.

Good posture refers not only to what we look like, but also reflects the strains it may be putting on certain parts of our body. The posture we have should make us feel comfortable, and able to move freely, and should not put undue stress on muscles or joints, and it should be automatically resumable after it has been displaced. Good posture results not only from the activity of a number of reflexes in the body, but also from our conscious effort to make certain muscles contract. This in turn is affected by a number of factors including how tired we are, our mood, and any discomfort, weight change, or muscle damage that may have occurred.

In the long term posture is important because incorrect posture leads to excess strain on joints and muscles which can lead to injury and discomfort. Good posture during pregnancy will help to prevent backache which is so common during pregnancy and afterwards.

The main postural changes that occur during pregnancy have been described on page 25.

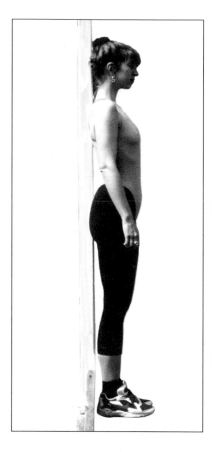

Checking upright posture

(FIGURE 6, LEFT)

Check your posture first of all by standing with your back against a wall, or look at yourself sideways in a mirror.

- There are normally two areas of curvature of the spine away from the wall.

- The first is at the neck, the second is in the lower back.

- These curves, and thus the gap between the back and the wall should be small.

- Pregnancy tends to pull the shoulders and the spine forwards, so exaggerating these curves.

HOW DO WE CORRECT POOR POSTURE?

- Stand with your back against the wall.

- Make sure your knees are relaxed, and feet slightly apart.

- Breathe in a relaxed slow manner.

- Try and straighten out the spine, aiming to press the lumbar curve, in the lower back, in towards the wall, by tucking your bottom in (forwards).

- At the same time, you should be tightening the abdominal muscles (effectively bringing the pelvis forwards slightly).

- Press your shoulders back towards the wall.

- Stretch your head high and feel your spine elongating.

Always remember

- Head high and neck tall
- Shoulders back and bottom tucked in - feel the contraction of the muscles running the length of the spine on either side
- Tummy held in
- Knees relaxed

Also, when standing, always stand with the weight of your body on both legs (not on one leg, as this leads to sideways curves in the spine and alters the relationship between the pelvis and the shoulder girdle).

Checking posture whilst sitting

(FIGURE 7A, RIGHT)

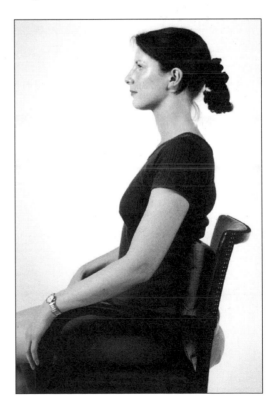

Posture when sitting is just as important as when standing. It is very easy to slump down when you are feeling tired into a soft sofa or chair and sit in a slouching position. Ideally, choose a chair that has a firm back and seat, and make sure that you sit well back into the chair. In this way your back will be held upright (sometimes a small pillow between the lower back and the back of the chair or sofa can help) and your knees will be relaxed.

Checking position whilst lying

This is not strictly to do with posture, but how we lie whilst pregnant can also have repercussions on our spine and other joints. Always try and lie on a firm mattress. Make sure that your spine is not twisted.

How to get up from a lying position

In the non-pregnant state, our abdominal muscles are very important when we sit up from the lying position. During pregnancy, the use of these muscles is greatly reduced because they are so stretched. Attempting to get up from the lying position, without the full use of the abdominal muscles, and with a heavy abdomen, can cause excessive strain to the spine.

THE BEST WAY OF GETTING UP FROM THE LYING POSITION
(FIGURES 7B AND 7C OPPOSITE)

- Bend your knees whilst pulling in your abdominal muscles.

- Roll over onto your side.

- Lever your upper body up with your arms.

- Swing your legs over the edge of the bed with knees together.

- Stand up.

This process should be reversed when lying down.

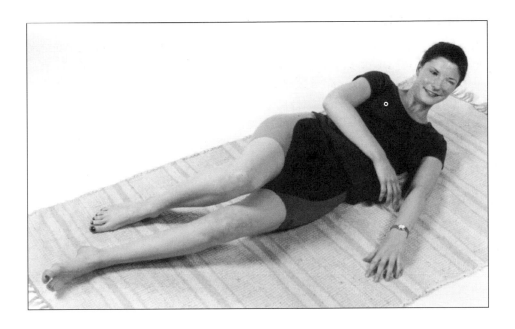

Figures 7b and 7c: Getting up from the lying position.

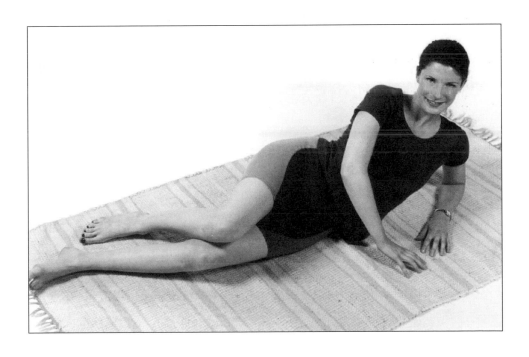

RELIEVING BACKACHE

Backache is common during pregnancy because of the strain of the ligaments and muscles between the bones of the spine and of the pelvis, and it is usually the result of the postural effects of pregnancy. It can cause local pain in any area from the neck and shoulders down to the lower back. Chronic back or neck pain of this sort can lead to muscle spasm, which can in turn lead to headaches and poor relaxation. Following the above guidelines may help to prevent the development of backache, and will certainly reduce its severity. If backache still occurs, however, the following approaches may help. Should severe backache develop, or if pain begins to radiate into the buttock or down into the legs, then a medical opinion should be sought.

The following exercises will help the different types of backache:

Neck and/or upper back and shoulder ache

- Slow neck turns

- Shoulder shrugs

- Shoulder circles

- Shoulder stretch

Lower backache

- Pelvic tilt whilst standing

- Pelvic circles whilst standing

- Pelvic pull up or 'bridging'

- Knee pull ups

Relieving neck and/or upper back and shoulder girdle ache

SLOW NECK TURNS
(FIGURE 8, BELOW)

This exercise uses the muscles at the front of the neck, and the paraspinals at the back. It may relieve muscle tension in the back of the neck and head.

- Stand with feet slightly apart, knees relaxed, and with good posture.

- Arms should hang loosely by your sides or rest on hips.

- Make sure your neck is stretched tall, and shoulders are back.

- Turn your head to the right (hold for count of 1 and') and left (hold for count of 2 and') slowly and with control.

- Turn the head only as far as is comfortable.

Repeat up to a count of 10.

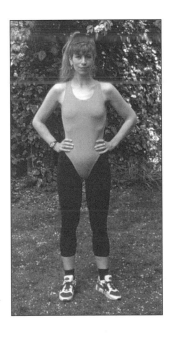 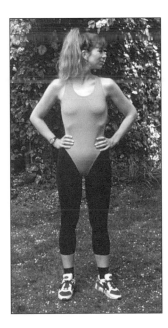 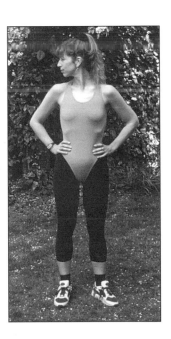

SHOULDER SHRUGS
(FIGURE 9, BELOW)

Strengthens the upper trapezius muscles and the muscles of the upper back. This exercise may help to relax the muscles in the neck and shoulders.

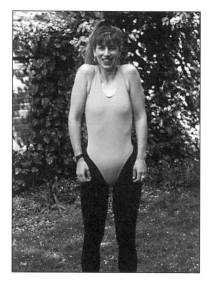

- Stand with feet slightly apart, arms hanging gently by your sides.

- Slowly raise your shoulders towards your ears, trying at the same time to push the shoulder blades towards each other in the midline of the back.

- The shoulders should then be gently released, slowly not suddenly, towards the resting position.

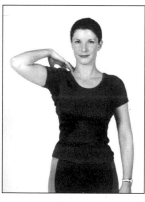

SHOULDER CIRCLES
(FIGURE 10, LEFT AND BELOW)

This strengthens the muscles of the shoulders and may help to relax these and the upper back muscles.

- Stand as for figure 9.

- Place hand gently cupped on the shoulders.

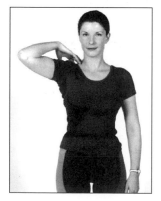

- Slowly rotate the elbow of the right arm forwards, out to the side, back and down.

- Repeat with the other arm then do both arms together.

Go through this sequence several times.

SHOULDER STRETCH
(FIGURE 11, BELOW)

This helps to relieve stiffness in the shoulders and upper back and chest.

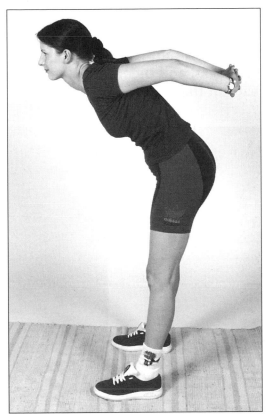

- Stand with correct posture, leaning slightly forwards from the hips.

- Clasp your hands together behind your back, or hold a short ribbon between them.

- Straighten your elbows out behind you and feel your chest stretch.

- Breathe normally a few times, then take a deep breath in and out.

- As you breathe out, bend forwards stretching your arms back and up as you go forwards.

Hold for a count of 4 then reverse the movements.

PELVIC PULL UP OR 'BRIDGING'
(FIGURE 14, BELOW)

This exercise tones the muscles of the abdomen, thighs and buttocks.

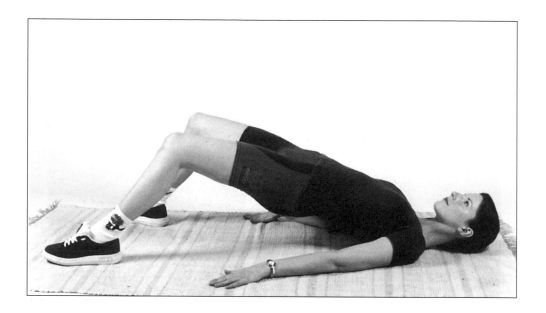

- Lie on your back with knees bent and feet placed on the floor slightly apart.

- Arms should be palm-down by your sides.

- Raise the hips off the floor and tighten your bottom as you do so.

- The pelvis should be higher than the navel, and the 'lift' should come from the pelvis rather than the waist.

Hold for a count of 5, breathing normally throughout, then reverse the movement gently.

KNEE PULL-UPS
(FIGURE 15, BELOW)

This may help to relieve lower back ache by unleashing the tension in muscles of the lower back and buttock.

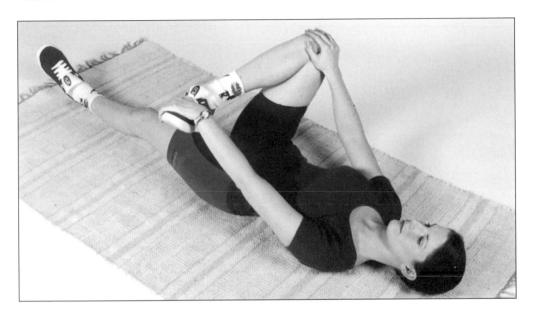

- Lie on your back with legs straight.

- Bend the right knee, and hold the knee with your right hand, and the ankle with your left.

- Pull the foot upwards in the direction of your navel

- Gradually pull the foot further as far as it will comfortably go in that direction.

- The other leg should be straight at all times, and the shoulders should remain on the floor as much as possible.

- Exercise of the right leg relieves right sided backache, and vice versa for the left.

Repeat several times, relaxing in between each pull-up.

RELAXATION

To relax means to 'loosen' or 'open up', to 'relieve the tension within'. Everyone needs to relax.

> **The stress of day-to-day life has many adverse effects on our bodies, such as**
>
> - Depletion of our energy stores
>
> - Increased levels of 'stress' and 'drive' hormones such as cortisol and adrenalin
>
> - Alterations in our metabolism
>
> - Alterations in our muscle activity
>
> - Excess stress can even affect the levels of our 'sex' hormones in such a way that the menstrual cycle can be altered

Relaxation is a way of relieving some of the effects of stress on our bodies, and is therefore probably of even more importance during pregnancy than it is at other times of life.

Relaxation can be found in many different guises. Some people find that a hobby or sport provides an antidote to the stresses of life; others find that meditation does the trick. True physical relaxation involves a releasing of the tension in muscles, and associated with this there may be an alteration in the heart beat, blood pressure and mental activity. It is the latter that the following regime aims to achieve. Unwinding mentally is often harder than learning how to relax your muscles. You may find that despite practicing these exercises, your mind continues to flood with thoughts but this tendency will decrease.

The ideal time to practice relaxation is at the end of a day, or after you have exercised. Here I outline two separate approaches to relaxation. The first is what is known as the 'contrast method' of relaxation which targets specific body parts. The second is based on Yoga methods which aim at relaxing both body and mind.

Practising contrast relaxation

The beauty of these exercises is that they can be done almost anywhere, and they can therefore be done whenever the relevant part of your body is feeling tense. The method is based on a strong contraction of muscle being followed by an equal relaxation of that muscle. The sequence of muscle contractions usually begins in the 'distal' part of the limb (eg the hand in the arm, the foot in the leg) and works inwards; ultimately, for example, the whole limb is contracted and then relaxed in reverse sequence. Alternatively, part of each exercise can be done.

CONTRAST RELAXATION FOR THE ARM
(TIGHTEN FOR COUNT OF 3, RELAX FOR COUNT OF 5)

- Make a fist, and let go.
- Bend the wrist backwards or forwards, and relax.
- Bend or straighten the elbow, and relax.
- Pull your elbow into your side, and relax.

Finally

- Tighten your fist, wrist, or elbow and let go in reverse order.

CONTRAST RELAXATION FOR THE LEG WHILST LYING ON BACK
(TIGHTEN FOR COUNT OF 3, RELAX FOR COUNT OF 5)

- Point your foot down, or pull foot up and let go (choose whichever position is least likely to give you cramp - usually pulling up).
- Straighten your knee slowly and tighten the thigh muscles; then let go.
- Tighten your buttocks then let go.

Finally

- Tighten the feet, knees and buttocks in sequence, then let go in reverse order.

CONTRAST RELAXATION FOR THE UPPER BODY AND HEAD
(TIGHTEN FOR COUNT OF 3, RELAX FOR COUNT OF 5)

This should be done whilst sitting comfortably in a firm padded chair with a high back providing a firm but comfortable support to your head and shoulders.

- Press your head against your support and let go.

- Press your shoulders against your support and let go.

Classic yoga relaxation

Ideally, this should be done in a quiet place away from bright lights and interruption. It is particularly useful at the end of the day, after an expedition, or when trying to get to sleep at night.

STAGE 1
(FIGURE 16, BELOW)

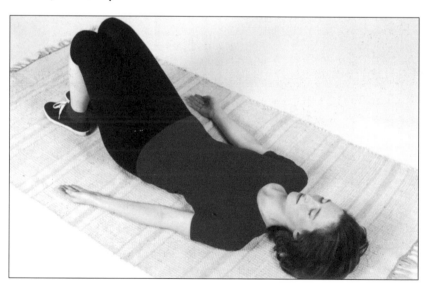

- Lie down on your back on a comfortable surface.

- Bend your knees and place your feet flat on the floor tucked up close to your bottom.

- Allow the muscles of your lower back and pelvis to relax so that the waist area moves down towards the floor.

- Straighten the curve of your neck, bringing your chin slightly forwards and down in the direction of your chest.

- Your throat should stay relaxed.

- Allow your eyes to close.

- Breathe out and let the tension in your shoulders go by allowing them to drop towards the floor.

- Let your arms and hands fall away from your body.

- The palms of your hands will face up towards the ceiling.

- Let the fingers of the hands curl naturally.

STAGE 2
(FIGURES 17A AND 17B, BELOW)

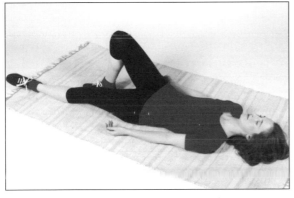 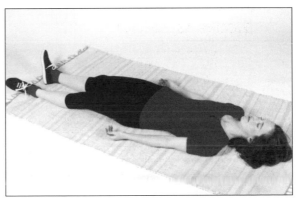

- Slowly straighten your legs out one by one.

- Let the legs roll outwards naturally with feet slightly apart.

- Breathe out and feel the whole weight of your body fall in towards the floor.

- Allow the quietness to come over your whole body.

- Relax the muscles of your face especially around the mouth and forehead.

- Breathe gently throughout, and as you do so, pause for a second at the end of each breath out, then allow the breath in to come of its own accord.

BREATHING

Breathing is important both during pregnancy and afterwards because it improves relaxation and expansion of the lungs. (Breathing exercises for use during labour will not be covered here.)

When we breathe normally, the breathing-in phase ('inspiration') is the active phase, whilst the breathing out phase ('expiration') is passive - in other words it occurs simply by relaxation of the muscles used during breathing in.

The muscles that control breathing are those of the rib cage, and those of the diaphragm. There are two types of normal breathing - shallow or quiet breathing, and deep breathing. Most of the time we breathe quietly. This involves the movement in and out of a relatively small amount of air, about 15 times per minutes (ie roughly 4 seconds per breath). So when doing deep breathing exercises, because the overall expansion of the chest is increased, the rate of breathing must be slower, so that hyperventilation does not occur.

Pregnant women have a tendency to hyperventilate (i.e. to breathe more quickly) partly because of the effects of certain hormones (eg progesterone) but also because the ability of the diaphragm to move down is reduced, and so breathing tends to be shallower.

Breathing correctly

Poor posture affects the way we breathe and the efficiency of breathing. Correct your posture first, as shown on page 70. Other factors that also affect our breathing patterns are tight, restrictive clothes and belts or bras that can restrict the expansion of the chest or descent of the diaphragm. Knowing how to correctly breathe quietly is important before attempting to practice deep breathing.

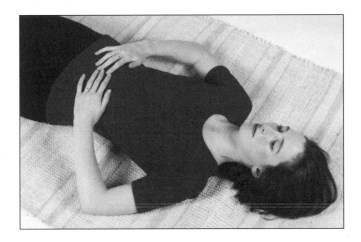

- Lie down on your back on the floor, and place the palms of your hands on your abdomen, fingers pointing towards the tummy button.

- As you breathe in, your hands will feel the movement of the abdomen beneath them. Any movement should be downwards - the abdomen should not push outwards or upwards (Figures 18a and 18b, above and below).

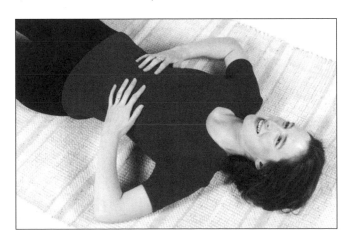

- In the same position, continue to move the hands upwards over your lower ribs.

- Now, as you breathe in the lower ribs should open out sideways, moving your hands apart as the chest expands (Figure 19, below).

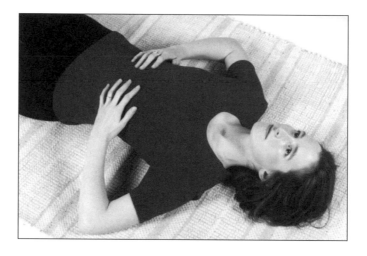

- Now move the hands high up on the upper chest with fingers and thumbs below the collar bones; here movement will be less because the inner ends of the ribs are fixed at this point.

- At the end of a deep breath in, you should feel an upward movement towards your hands (Figure 20, below).

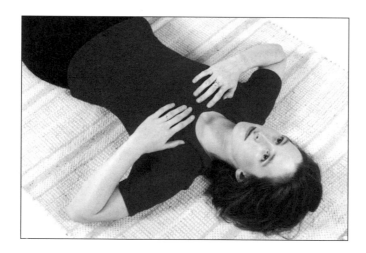

Deep breathing

This can be very relaxing, and is useful to practice simply as an exercise to improve your breathing. Once you are satisfied that you breathe correctly, you can move on to deep breathing. Deep breathing can be done lying or sitting, or in whichever position you feel comfortable.

Practicing deep breathing

- Allow your breathing pattern to become quiet and even.

- Breathe out beyond the point where you would normally stop.

- As you come to the end of your breath, pause for a second.

- Then begin to breathe in slowly and deeply.

- Your shoulders, throat and neck should be relaxed.

- Breathe out slowly.

This kind of breathing may make you feel you are suffocating at the beginning. If so, try only one breath at a time, followed by a few normal breaths. If you feel like yawning, you may need to increase the speed of the out-and-in breath.

Once you feel comfortable, you can increase the number of 'deep breaths' that are done sequentially. After a period of deep breathing, you should be still for a while before moving around again. You should feel relaxed.

During these breathing exercises, take care not to 'hyperventilate' - this can cause lightheadedness and tingling of the fingertips and mouth area.

PELVIC FLOOR EXERCISES

Pelvic floor exercises are important because they improve the tone of the muscles of the perineum and pelvic floor and sphincters (see p22), and help to repair damaged muscles. These exercises have also been demonstrated to be one of the most effective ways of helping wounds or tears heal after childbirth.

The beauty of these exercises is that they can be done whenever you remember, and no one can tell you are doing them! Although these exercises are introduced here, they are perhaps particularly important after pregnancy, and the presence of perineal stitches should not prevent you from doing them. Exercises like this tend to improve the blood supply to the perineum, and so help the healing process. They also help to relieve discomfort.

There are basically two parts of your body that you must become familiar with controlling: the pelvic floor and the sphincters. The sphincters are the rings of muscle that encircle the urethra (the opening from which the urine comes) and the anus. These sphincters are situated within the muscles of the pelvic floor. The function of the pelvic floor and sphincters has been described on pages 26-27. Control of the sphincters in every day life normally occurs almost without thinking; but in fact we have very accurate voluntary control of these rings of muscle.

- For the urinary sphincter, so that you get to know what controlling it feels like, try stopping and starting the stream whilst you are in the middle of urinating. Once you have got the feeling of this control, this exercise can be repeated throughout the day, preferably when you are not passing urine.

- Contractions of the muscles forming the anal sphincter can best be felt when you are trying to stop yourself opening your bowels. This muscle contraction is often accompanied by elevation of some of the other pelvic floor muscles. Muscles of the pelvic floor proper, as well as the muscles surrounding the entry to the vagina, are often contracted when we attempt to contract the sphincters.

- Contraction of the muscles surrounding the opening to the vagina can best be practiced during sexual intercourse, by trying to grip your partner's penis. Tightening the muscles of the sphincters and, at the same time trying to draw all the muscles upward into the pelvis is the most effective way of exercising the muscles of the pelvic floor.

In addition to the aforementioned exercises, specific pelvic floor exercises include the following which can be done standing, lying or sitting. Throughout these exercises, breathe gently and try not to hold your breath.

PULLING UP AND LETTING GO

- Draw up the muscles of the pelvic floor and tighten the sphincters for a count of 2 seconds, then release fully.

- On releasing, push very gently so that you can feel the vagina opening a little. Do this several times a day.

LIFTING AND HOLDING

- Draw up the pelvic floor in 3 stages, stopping and holding momentarily at each stage.

- With each upward contraction, try to pull the floor of muscles higher and higher.

- On releasing, relax the muscles gently downwards. Never push down hard especially if you have had stitches to the perineum.

AQUA-EXERCISE

Swimming is a favourite exercise of mine, and during pregnancy this can provide an excellent answer to a number of potential problems. Of all sports and exercise programmes, it is the only one that I can whole-heartedly recommend for all stages of pregnancy. In the earlier stages of pregnancy it is also the exercise I would recommend for those women who wish to exercise with the aim of improving aerobic capacity.

Swimming is an excellent sport as it exercises practically every muscle group in the body. It is non-weight bearing and so causes minimal damage to the joints. It involves spending much of the time in the near-horizontal position which improves circulation in the legs. Swimming is also relaxing and can relieve muscle tensions. It supports you and the weight of your baby whilst at the same time enabling you to exercise. Swimming is a powerful muscle strengthener, and will prepare you well for the demanding task of labour and childbirth. Finally, swimming involves controlled and deep breathing which will be of use during labour.

Safety tips for swimming whilst pregnant

- Remember that pool sides can be slippery, and you are more liable to fall when pregnant.

- Use the steps or ladder to get in or out, or, if you are used to doing so, slip in gently off the edge of the pool.

- Do not swim if your waters have broken. If you feel them breaking whilst swimming, get out of the pool at once to reduce the risk of infection.

- Swimming itself poses no additional infection risks to pregnant women provided the pool is well-chlorinated. There is no evidence that chlorine itself in the doses used in pools is of any harm.

- Avoid swimming if the pool is crowded - this increases the chances of being kicked or jumped upon.

- Do not dive or jump into the water. Stop swimming if you feel excessively tired, faint, or feel any discomfort.

Standard swimming

If you are someone who swims regularly anyway, then continuing to swim during pregnancy will seem natural. As with all forms of exercise, swimming should only be done at a level your body is accustomed to, and during pregnancy, this level will alter as your body metabolism changes, and as your centre of gravity alters.

If you are unaccustomed to swimming regularly, it is best to make a gentle start, swimming for short periods once or twice a week. This can be gradually built up during pregnancy so that you may be going as often and 3 or 4 times towards the end of pregnancy. However, the nature of the swimming should alter with pregnancy. To begin with, you should be able to swim much as you did before pregnancy. After six weeks you may be feeling more tired than usual, and your exercise capacity may change. Never swim or exercise to the extent that you feel drained.

During the last stages of pregnancy the sheer bulk of the abdomen will limit your abilities to perform different swimming strokes.

Swimming strokes

BREAST STROKE

This is probably the swimming stroke best suited to all stages of pregnancy. It can be taken gently and you can see where you are going. It should be avoided if you have backache as there is a tendency to arch the lower back whilst doing breast stroke which can aggravate backache. As pregnancy advances, it is more difficult to keep your legs as horizontal behind you as before, so let them hang down a little more vertically.

FRONT CRAWL

A little more difficult to manage in later pregnancy, because the weight of the abdomen tends to pull your body vertically, and the arm movements in front crawl are less effective than those in breast stroke at keeping your body level.

BACK STROKE
This is excellent because it tones the upper arms and chest muscles, especially the pectorals, and is also very good for the abdominal muscles.

BUTTERFLY
This is not a stroke that many people can manage, but there is no reason why this should not be continued during early pregnancy if it is a stroke you are familiar with. During pregnancy, the problems for managing the stroke are as for front crawl.

All swimming strokes are good, general strengtheners for the muscles of the arms, legs, buttocks and back.

If you are not a 'swimmer' but would like to take advantage of all the other benefits that exercise in water can offer, you may find that your local pool runs an Aquanatal class. If not, or if you prefer to do your own, then I suggest the following series of exercises:

- Pool edge exercises
- Shallow end exercises
- Arm exercises
- Leg exercises
- Waist exercises
- Abdominal exercises

These will be explained on the following pages.

Shaping Up

The following exercises are to be done in the pool

Before getting into the pool, sit on the edge, and dangle your feet in the water. Circle your feet at the ankles several times in each direction. Next, alternatively point and pull up your toes at the ankles several times.

Shallow end exercises

These exercises should be performed standing in waist deep water.

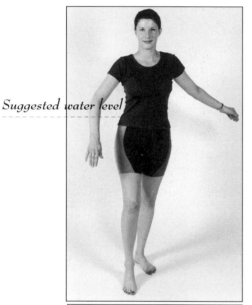

Suggested water level

WALKING WARM UP
(FIGURE 21, LEFT)

- Walk slowly through the water for 60 seconds, using your arms like oars, and paddling the water with the palms of your hands.

This exercise is good for all the muscles of the arms, legs and buttocks.

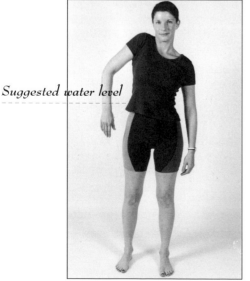

Suggested water level

SHOULDER LIFTS
(FIGURE 22, LEFT)

- Remembering your posture, slowly raise your right shoulder up towards the right ear and hold for a count of 2, then lower it again.

Repeat several times and then switch to the other shoulder. This exercise is good for the upper shoulder muscles.

Arm exercises

HORIZONTAL ARM STOKES

(FIGURES 23A AND 23B, BELOW)

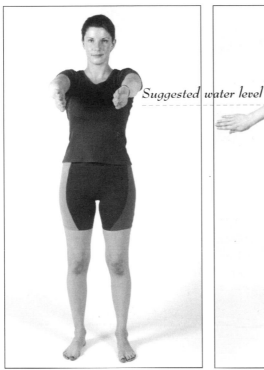
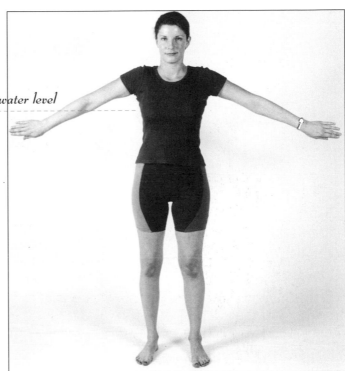

Suggested water level

- Move into slightly deeper water, so that your arms are covered with water.

- Lift your arms out in front of you with palms facing outwards.

- Slowly move the arms horizontally outwards from the centre through the water, so that the arms are acting like big paddles.

- When the arms are stretched out to each side, turn the palms of the hands in the opposite direction (i.e. facing inwards), and reverse the direction of movement.

Repeat several times.

Waist exercises

UPPER BODY TURNS
(FIGURES 24A AND 24B, BELOW)

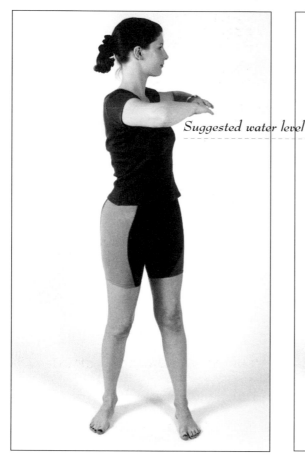
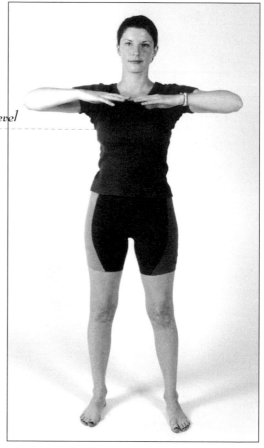

Suggested water level

- Stand with the arms bent at the elbows, held horizontally, with fingers pointing towards each other.

- Slowly rotate the upper part of your body 90 degrees to the right, over a count of '3' and back to the centre.

Repeat several times, and then an equal number of times to the left.

Leg exercises

SINGLE LEG PULL-UPS
FIGURES 25 AND 26, BELOW)

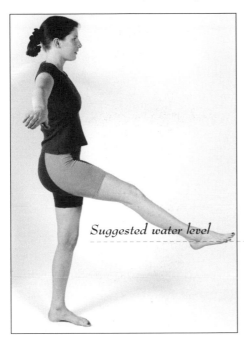
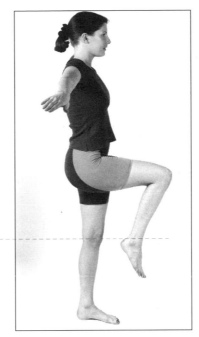

Suggested water level

- Move to the edge of the pool at the shallow end, and stand with your back against the side of the pool.

- Stretch your arms out to the sides and grip the bar or edge of the pool.

- Pull the right knee slowly up towards your chest whilst the left foot is on the floor of the pool.

- Straighten out the right leg in front of you, pull up the toes of the foot at the ankle, then point your toe and then relax.

- Draw the knee back in towards your chest, and place the foot on the floor of the pool.

Repeat this sequence several times with the right leg, and then follow with the left.

Abdominal exercises

TWO LEG PULL-UPS

- Using the same position as figure 25, this time try and lift both knees slowly up towards your chest.

- Stretch both legs out in front of you, pull back the toes of both feet, then point the toes.

- Next, bend the knees again as you draw the legs back in towards your chest.

- Finally lower the legs to the floor of the pool.

This exercise is excellent for the abdominal muscles, and the muscles running the length of the spine (these are involved in the 'uncurling' process as the legs are straightened out again as they return to the floor).

These exercises will help to prepare you for labour and will improve your muscle strength and fitness. By the time it comes to labour you should be very used to performing pelvic floor exercises, you should find it easier to relax and the control of your breathing should have improved. All this will greatly help you during the birth process and afterwards.

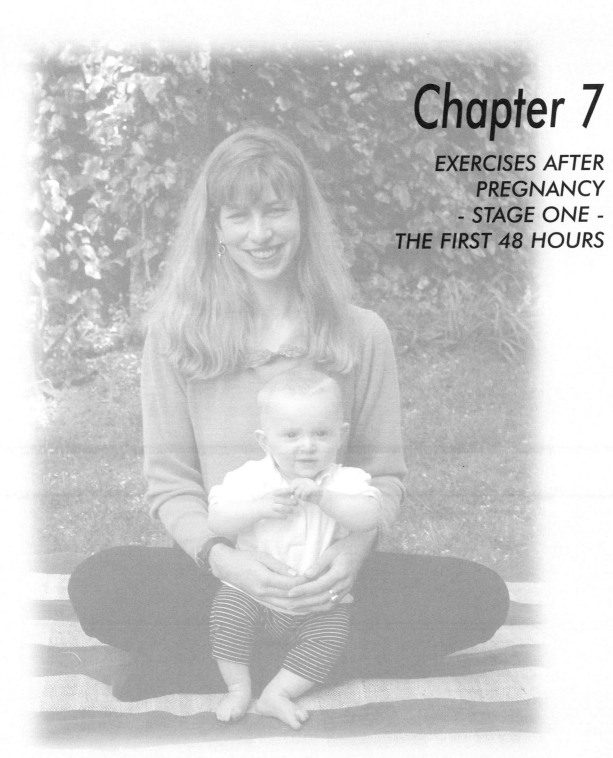

Chapter 7

EXERCISES AFTER
PREGNANCY
- STAGE ONE -
THE FIRST 48 HOURS

In the first few days after birth, you may feel exhilarated at the presence of your new baby, but you will also almost certainly feel very tired both physically and mentally, depending on how often you are woken up by your baby! Therefore for the first 2 weeks especially with a first baby, most mothers are not yet ready to start a proper exercise routine.

For your exercises you are going to require an interruption-free period of about 40 minutes, and such a period will emerge once your baby has settled into a routine of his/her own. It helps if someone can look after the baby whilst you do your exercises.

If you have had a vaginal delivery, you may be sore in the perineal area, especially if there has been a tear or if you have needed an episiotomy with stitches. You may also be getting some 'afterpains' which result from contraction of the uterus. This is usually most pronounced when breast feeding, when the hormone oxytocin is released. Afterpains can also occur if the lower abdomen is rubbed. After pains are basically a good sign that the uterus is contracting and shrinking back towards its pre-pregnant state. Using the breathing exercises will help if the pains are distressing.

SAFETY ASPECTS AFTER PREGNANCY

The abdominal muscles will be lax and flabby. In addition, the two bands of rectus muscle that run down the middle of the abdomen will not yet have come together in the midline. Great care, therefore, must be taken to follow the guidelines described in Chapter 5. In particular, do not attempt any exercise that is too strenuous as this will strain the lax muscles. During this period, any movement may result in a small amount of discharge or blood appearing from the vagina. This is normal (heavy blood or discharge is not normal, and if this occurs, you should seek medical attention), and should not inhibit you from exercising.

Carrying and holding your baby

New born babies are not heavy and many babies do enjoy being held and carried much of the time by their mothers! This activity on its own will help to build the strength in your arms and upper body. There are several ways in which a baby can be held and carried. Remember the baby's head will need to be supported in all positions in the early weeks. Follow the basic guidelines about moving and standing described in chapter 5, so as to avoid back strain.

Suggestions about how to carry your baby

- A baby can be held upright, supported by the crook of one arm over the bottom, and the other arm holding the baby's head and upper body, with the baby's front against your chest, and head peering over your shoulder. This is also a good position for winding the baby.

- A baby can be held in one arm, the baby's back held against your abdomen, and the arm fixing the baby over the shoulder with a hand holding the baby between the legs. Your forearm will thus rest over the baby's abdomen, and his/her head will rest in the crook of your arm.

- A baby can be held and carried in a sling or baby-pouch. It is definitely worth getting one that is the right size for your small baby, rather than a larger one which the baby will 'grow into', as they are more likely to be able to see out of a smaller one!

EXERCISES FOR THE FIRST 48 HOURS

For women who have had a vaginal delivery

Both pelvic floor exercises and the breathing and relaxation exercises can be practiced whilst lying in bed and should be done as often as you like. They are not tiring and help to speed your recovery, improve blood circulation and prepare you for more demanding exercises later on.

With all of the exercises, the more often you do them, the quicker your recovery will be. Do remember to wear a supportive bra.

In order to monitor your progress over the next few weeks, you can make some initial measurements:

- Measure your waist at the level of the navel.

- Measure the circumference of the tops of your arms and thighs.

- Measure the gap between the rectus muscles (see opposite).

Pelvic floor exercise

Do the pelvic floor exercises described on page 90 as often as you can.

Breathing and relaxation exercises

The exercises shown in Chapter 6, pages 87-89 can be done as often as you like.

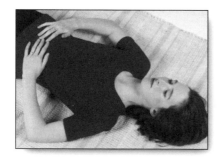

Early abdominal exercises

CHECKING THE RECTUS MUSCLES
(FIGURE 27, BELOW)

Immediately after delivery, most women will have a gap of some degree between the two muscles. In many women this is around three finger breadths wide, but in some it will be as much as four or five. First, make a check of how far apart the rectus muscles are. This is done by lying on your back on a flat surface with your knees bent.

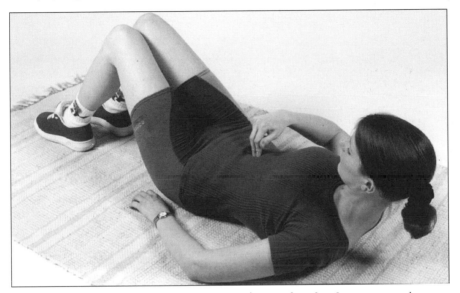

Figure 27: Checking the gap between the two bands of rectus muscle

- The gap between the muscles will not be felt when the muscles are relaxed, so the only way to test for it is by contracting the rectus muscles.

- Place the fingers of the right hand just above the navel.

- The left arm is placed down by your side.

- Gently lift your head and shoulders up off the floor or bed.

- You will feel the two edges of the rectus muscle contract at the edges of your fingers.

Exercising the abdominal muscles

EARLY CURL-UPS
(FIGURE 28, BELOW)

This exercise strengthens the rectus muscles and helps to close the gap between them.

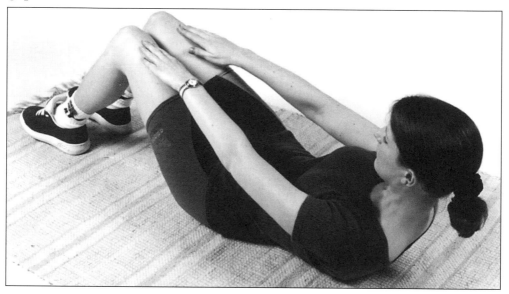

- Lie on your back with knees bent and arms resting on your thighs.

- With your chin tucked into your chest, gently lift up your head and shoulders off the floor or bed, a few inches, sliding your arms towards the knees.

- Lie back again slowly. The upward movement should be done whilst breathing out, and the downward movement whilst breathing in.

Do it 3 or 4 times initially and build up to 10.

PELVIC TILT
(FIGURE 12, RIGHT, SEE PAGE 78)

If you have a very firm bed, this exercise can be done in bed. Otherwise it can be done whilst standing. It strengthens the abdominal and back muscles, as well as toning the buttocks.

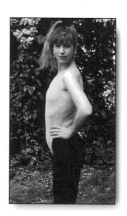

Leg exercises

SIDE LEG LIFTS

(FIGURES 29A AND 29B, BELOW) - ABDUCTORS

This exercise is good for the muscles of the outer side of the thigh (the abductor muscles) and the buttock. It also helps to strengthen the abdominal muscles as these need to be braced throughout the leg movements.

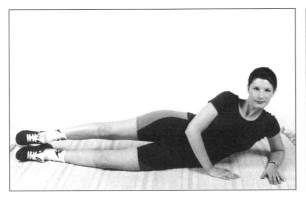 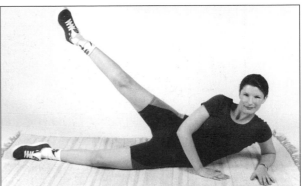

- Lie on your left side with your left forearm resting on the floor at right angles to your body.

- An alternative position is leaning on the left elbow, with the head resting in the palm of your hand.

- The right hand should be placed palm down in front of your chest.

- Make sure the plane of your body is at right angles to the floor.

- Bend the left (lowermost) leg slightly at the knee, and start the exercise with the right foot touching the floor.

- Lift the right leg with the knee straight as far off the floor as you can, and then lower it slowly back to the floor, but not quite touching the floor.

- Make sure that the hips are level one above the other, and that you are not leaning forwards or heavily into the lower arm and shoulder.

Repeat a few times then change to the other side.

FOOT EXERCISES IN BED
(FIGURES 30A AND 30B, BELOW)
These are especially good for improving the circulation in the legs, as they exercise the muscles of the calf which helps to 'pump' blood back towards the heart. They can be done as often as you like, and when lying or sitting.

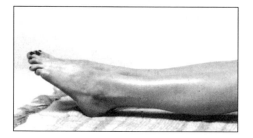 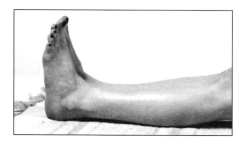

- Lie on your back with legs straight out in front of you.

- With both feet, point your toes and bend the foot downwards as much as possible, for a count of 2.

- This should be quickly followed by a full upward movement, 'un-pointing' the toes as you go.

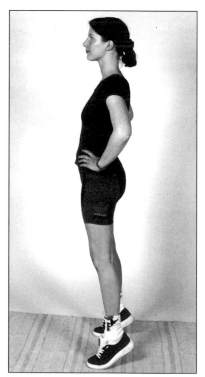

FOOT EXERCISES WHILST STANDING
(FIGURE 31, LEFT)
This exercise helps to reduce swelling in the ankles, and improve circulation in the lower legs.

- Stand with your feet slightly apart and hands on hips.

- Lift yourself up onto the ball of your feet, hold for 3 and lower.

Repeat these exercises several times a day.

EXERCISES FOR WOMEN WHO HAVE HAD A CAESAREAN SECTION

After the operation there may be pain over the incision as well as afterpains. The abdominal muscles will be lax and this will be further compromised by the fact that there has been a surgical incision through them. You may feel very sore every time you move to sit up or turn.

Lying down

For general comfort, women who have had a caesarean section may find that whilst sitting in bed, you are best supported by several pillows whilst lying in the semi-reclining position.

Getting in and out of bed

- When getting in and out of bed, use your hands to help push you up from the lying position.

- Sidle your bottom to the edge of the bed and place both feet firmly on the floor.

- Push yourself up with your feet, whilst holding the lower abdomen over the incision with your hands.

- You may need help with getting up in the first few days.

- When getting back into bed, move towards it so that the backs of your knees are firmly pressed against the bed, and you are close to the head of the bed.

- Lower yourself down using your hands to help if necessary, so that your bottom lands close to the centre of the bed.

- Lift your legs one at a time onto the bed, using hands if necessary, and lie back.

An alternative approach is to use the method described in Chapter 6, page 73, 'How to get up from a lying position'.

Standing and walking

Standing and walking can be awkward as many women are afraid to 'stretch' the wound. It may help with this feeling if you hold the wound firmly with one hand as you straighten up. Try to stand straight, remembering all the tips about posture!

Women who have had a caesarean section will probably lag behind other mothers who have had vaginal births, by about 2 weeks, in terms of exercise and physical capacity. The exercises shown in Chapter 8 should therefore only be begun once the incision has healed properly, and once you feel comfortable enough to do them.

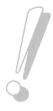

> **If you are in any doubt about your ability to carry out these exercises safely, consult your doctor.**

EXERCISES FOR THE FIRST 48 HOURS

The following exercises can be done straight away, and will aid healing and help you to relax, as well as improve the circulation in your legs:

CONTRAST RELAXATION EXERCISES FOR ARMS AND LEGS, HEAD AND NECK
(PAGES 83-84)

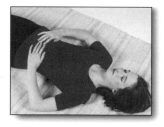

BREATHING EXERCISES
(PAGE 87)

PELVIC FLOOR EXERCISES
(PAGES 90-92)

Even if you have not had a vaginal birth, there is still extra fluid and congestion in the perineal area and the exercises help the blood to circulate and any swelling to subside.

FOOT EXERCISES IN BED
(FIGURES 30A AND 30B, RIGHT, PAGE 108)

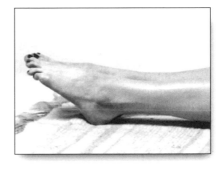

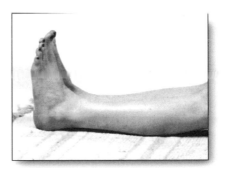

BUTTOCK SQUEEZE

- Lie on your back with knees straight. Rhythmically squeeze and relax the cheeks of your bottom together, whilst at the same time drawing up your pelvic floor during the squeezing phase.

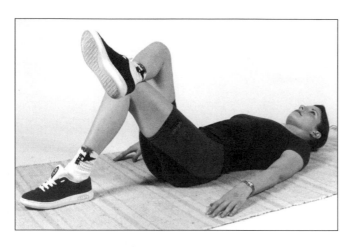

ANKLE CIRCLES
(FIGURES 32A AND 32B, LEFT AND BELOW)

- Lie on your back with both knees bent and feet flat on the floor.

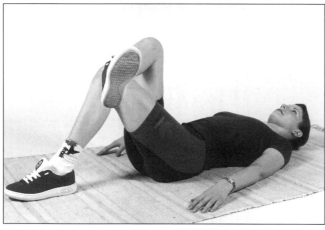

- Raise one leg and place the calf across the other knee (crossing the legs in this way should be avoided unless you are at the same time exercising the calf muscles as in this exercise).

- Rotate the ankle in as wide and sweeping a circular movement as possible in one direction.

Repeat the required number of times and then reverse directions.

These exercises should be continued until you are ready to move on to the exercises shown in the next section: this may take up to two weeks. Normally this takes two to three days. In addition to the above exercises, in the early days after birth, try and begin to be as generally active as you can, without causing excess tiredness or strain.

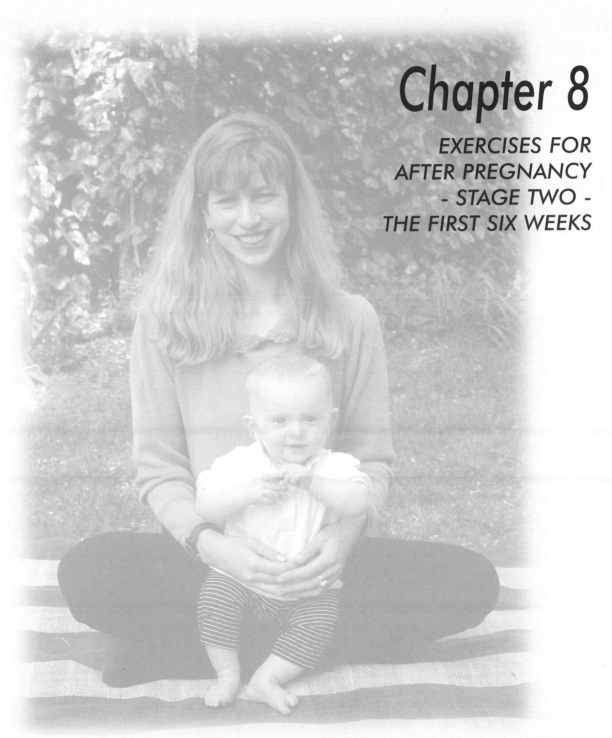

Chapter 8

EXERCISES FOR
AFTER PREGNANCY
- STAGE TWO -
THE FIRST SIX WEEKS

CHECKLIST

A: Standing Exercises

- Shoulder shrugs
- Chest hugs
- Elbow squeeze
- Hip presses and diagonal trunk bends
- Quarter waist turns
- High knee lifts

B: Chair Exercises

- Forward leg lifts
- Easy side leg lifts
- Waist twists
- Thigh rotations
- Controlled squats

C: Dumb Bell Exercises

- Shoulder girdle
- Alternating bicep curls
- Double tricep kick-backs
- Single arm extensions
- Double arm extensions
- Waist side-bends
- Forward lunges

D: *Floor Exercises*

- Bottom and adductor squeeze
- Knee waist turns
- Centre curl-ups

  Stage 2
  Stage 3

- Diagonal curl-ups

  Stage 2
  Stage 3

- Leg scissors
- Ankle circles
- Side leg lifts
- Head and shoulder lifts
- Backward leg lifts

THIS IS WHERE YOU REALLY START TO SHAPE UP!

Exactly when in the 6 weeks following birth you begin this programme depends on how you are coping with the arrival of the new baby, and on how tired you are. ***Do not try to start before you feel ready.*** You will need to find a suitable period each day to do the exercises. Whilst this requires some degree of organisation and determination, it is really worth setting aside the time to do them.

Many mothers manage to do the exercises with the baby watching. This sometimes results in frequent interruption, so I suggest you ensure that someone can care for your baby for the short time that it takes to do the exercises. That will enable you to concentrate fully on yourself, and to ensure that the exercises are done correctly. Obviously, mothers who have had a caesarean section will need to be absolutely sure that their wound has healed and that there are no medical or obstetric complications before they start the exercises.

> **Whenever you begin this series of exercises, make sure that you do them for at least 6 weeks before moving on to the more demanding programme shown in the next chapter. In the first few weeks it is important also to ensure that you get adequate rest especially if you are breast feeding. Remember to do the pelvic floor exercises and posture checks as often as you can.**

The following exercises are aimed at muscle toning and strengthening. They take about 35 minutes to complete. Try to do the whole routine at least two to three times per week, more often if you are able. However just once a week is better than nothing at all! As the weeks go on, you will get to know the exercises better and you will soon find you can do the routine without referring to the book. By the end of the 6 weeks you should be ready to move on to the exercises shown in Chapter 9.

SECTION 1

The Warm Up

This is done whilst standing. Start with feet slightly apart. Make sure the room is not too warm, and that you are well hydrated before you start. If you are breast feeding it is more comfortable if you have breastfed your baby before starting the exercises.

DO A POSTURE CHECK

(FIGURE 6, RIGHT, PAGE 70)

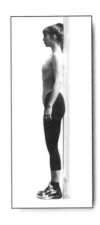

PELVIC FLOOR EXERCISES X 3

(PAGES 90-92)

SLOW NECK TURNS X 5 TO EACH SIDE

(FIGURE 8, BELOW, PAGE 75)

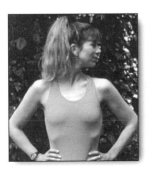
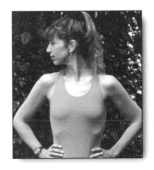

ARM CIRCLES X 10 FORWARDS AND 10 BACKWARDS
(FIGURES 33A AND 33B, BELOW)

This exercise strengthens all the muscles of the shoulder girdle and also the pectoral muscles in the front of the chest. They also help to relieve tightness in these muscles and stiffness in the shoulders.

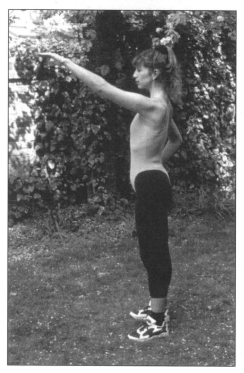 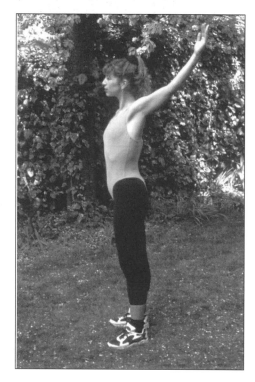

FORWARDS

- Stand with feet slightly apart, knees relaxed.

- Make sure your bottom and tummy are tucked in.

- Start with arms by your sides, hands relaxed.

- Swing your arms slowly backwards, then out to the sides, up past your ears, forward and then down.

- The entire movement should be slow, not forced and should not cause any discomfort.

BACKWARDS

- The forward movement is reversed.

SIDE BENDS X 10 EACH SIDE
(FIGURES 34A AND 34B, BELOW)

This exercise strengthens and tones all the muscles on each side of the abdomen and also those running the length of the spine.

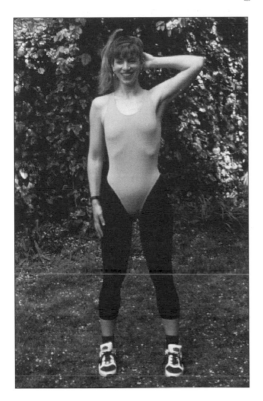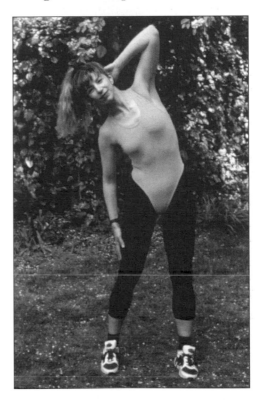

- Stand with feet slightly apart.

- Place one hand on the side of your head, and the other on the outer aspect of the upper thigh on the other side.

- Slowly bend down sideways.

- Run the hand down the outer aspect of the thigh and calf as far down towards the ankle as you can.

- Reverse up the thigh, move through the upright centre position, and repeat to the other side.

- The movements should be slow and unforced. Only bend as far as you feel comfortable.

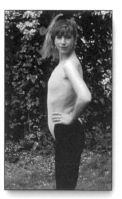

PELVIC TILT X 10
(FIGURE 12, LEFT, PAGE 78)

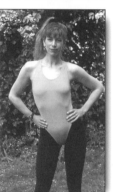

PELVIC CIRCLES X 10 EACH DIRECTION
(FIGURE 13, LEFT, PAGE 79)

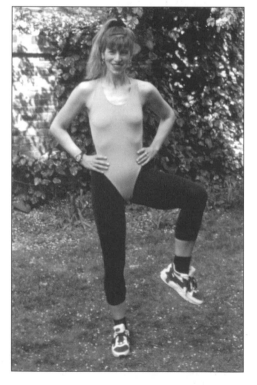

LOW KNEE LIFTS X 10 EACH LEG
(FIGURE 35, BOTTOM LEFT)

This exercise uses the muscles that run along the spine, abdominal muscles, buttock and thigh muscles.

- Check posture.

- Stand with feet slightly apart, hands on waist.

- Lift one leg with knee bent and turned slightly out to the side, and toes of that foot pointed, up to the level of the navel.

- Lower the foot to the ground by reversing the movement. Through-out, the shoulders should be level, and back upright.

Repeat and then move to the other leg.

SECTION 2 *Muscle Toning And Strengthening*
A: Standing exercises

SHOULDER SHRUGS X 10
(FIGURE 9, RIGHT, PAGE 76)

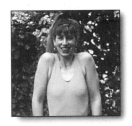

CHEST HUGS X 10
(FIGURES 36A AND 36B, BELOW)
This exercise is excellent for the pectoral muscles at the front of the chest and also for the muscles in the upper part of the back and around the shoulder blades.

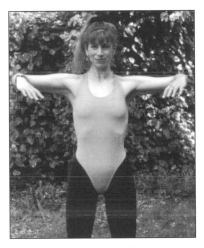 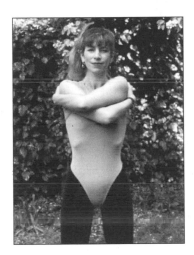

- Stand with feet slightly apart.

- Bend your arms at the elbow and also slightly at the wrists.

- Hold them out to the side, almost horizontal, slightly below shoulder height.

- Rotate the arms slowly, and bring them together, allowing the hands to cross each other, until they grasp the opposite shoulder blade.

The movement is then reversed, this time bringing the elbows as far out to the sides as is comfortable. Repeat the exercise, alternating which arm is uppermost.

HIP PRESSES AND DIAGONAL UPPER BODY BENDS X 10 EACH SIDE
(FIGURES 37A AND 37B, BELOW)

This exercise uses the muscles of the buttocks (hip press section) and all the muscles of the abdomen on each side of the body.

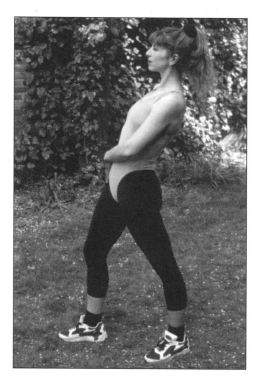 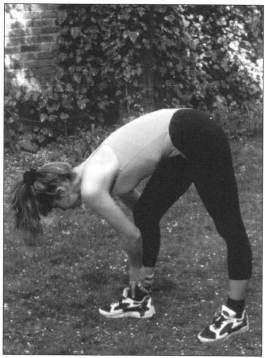

- Stand with one foot slightly in front of the other and toes pointing forwards.

- Make sure the knees are 'soft' and not pressed back.

- Place both hands on the front of the thigh of the foot that is in front.

- Bend forwards slowly towards the front foot, running the hands down the leg as far as is comfortable.

- Come back up in reverse direction, and as you return to the upright position, tilt the hip forwards, tightening the buttock muscles as you do so.

Continue on the same side for the required number, then change position and repeat on the other side.

B: Floor Exercises

An introduction to 'curl-ups'

These exercises are very important for strengthening your abdomen and restoring your waist line. Strong abdominal muscles also help with posture. The safety guidelines described in Chapter 5 should be followed.

Here I have used two types of sit up exercise. The first (centre curl-ups) are especially aimed at the rectus muscles, whilst the second (diagonal curl-ups) work on the oblique muscles of the abdomen. For both centre and diagonal curl-ups, there are 3 stages according to their difficulty. Some women will find the third stage too difficult even after several weeks, but with continued practice most women should be able to do them.

Some general advice about curl-ups

- **In all sit-up exercises you should breathe out as you come up and breathe in as you lie back down.**

- **The lying down section is as important as the sitting up part, and should be equally well controlled.**

- **Never fall or slump heavily back onto the surface.**

- **Curl-ups should never be done with the feet held down, or with the head pulled forwards by hands clasped behind the neck.**

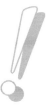

FOR ALL THESE START WITH 5 AND INCREASE TO 10 WHEN READY

CENTRE CURL-UPS
(FIGURE 38, BELOW)

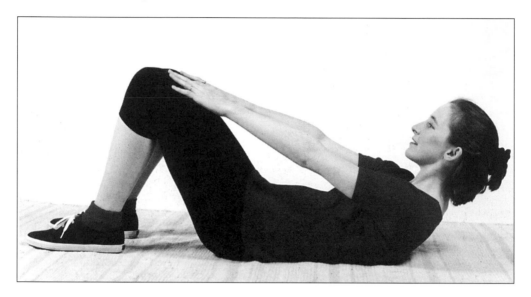

- Lie on your back on a flat, firm, comfortable surface.

- Knees should be bent with feet flat on floor.

If you have separation of the rectus muscles of 2 finger breadths or more, you should cross your arms over your abdomen, holding the opposite side of the waist in with each hand. If the separation is not greater than 2 fingerbreadths, proceed as follows:

- Rest both hands on the fronts of your thighs.

- As you breathe out, lift your head and shoulders up off the floor attempting to look at your knees.

- Hold for a count of 3 and then return slowly to the flat position, breathing in as you do so.

Repeat.

DIAGONAL CURL-UPS
(FIGURE 39, BELOW)

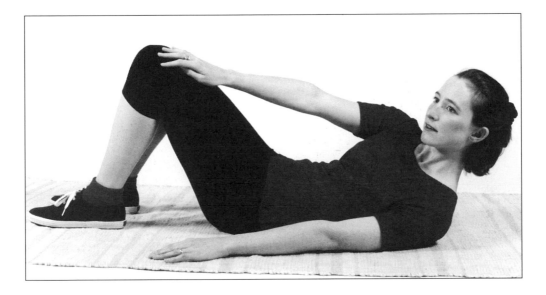

- Basic position is as for centre curl-ups except that one hand (say the left to start with) is resting on the floor by your side.

- The other hand (right in this case) should be placed on the front of the opposite (left) thigh.

- Then raise the right shoulder and head off the floor whilst at the same time sliding the right hand up the left thigh, attempting to touch the left knee.

- Return slowly to the starting position, and repeat with the other side.

Repeat this pair of diagonal curl-ups as required.

BOTTOM AND ADDUCTOR SQUEEZE

(FIGURES 40A AND 40B THIS PAGE. FIGURES 40C, 40B AND 40A, OPPOSITE)
This exercise is excellent for the gluteal muscles of the bottom and for the abductors - the muscles running along the inner aspect of the thighs. It is also good for the pelvic floor muscles.

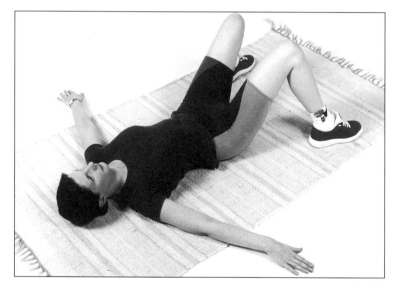

- Lie on your back with knees bent and feet placed flat on the floor, slightly further apart than your hips.

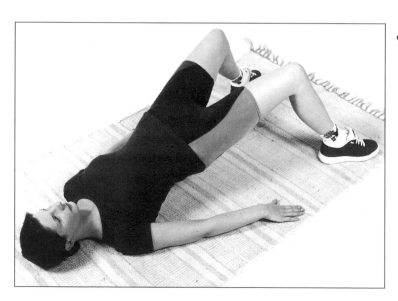

- Rhythmically squeeze in your buttocks at the same time as tilting the pelvis off the floor (this should result in the arch of your lower back becoming 'uncurved', at the same time as lifting the bottom off the floor).

- Once you reach the height of the movement, squeeze your thighs together (bringing the knees together too), and tighten the pelvic floor muscles. Imagine that you have a big beach ball between your legs which you are gripping hard.

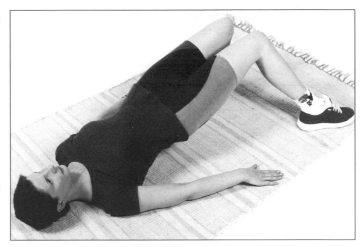

- Reverse the movements by first bringing the legs apart from the knees and the inner thighs.

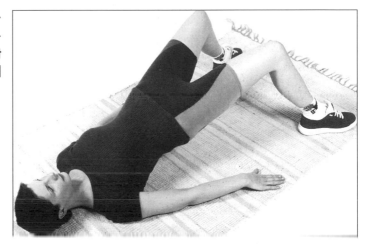

- Finally, relax the buttock and return the lower spine to its normal curvature.

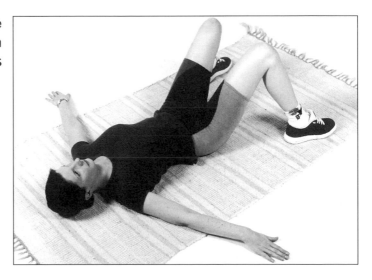

ANKLE CIRCLES X 10 EACH DIRECTION WITH EACH FOOT
(FIGURES 32A AND 32B, BELOW, PAGE 112)

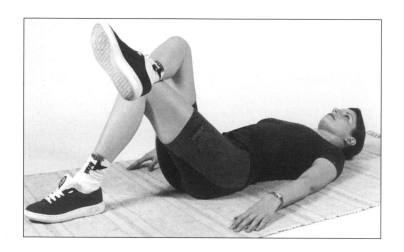

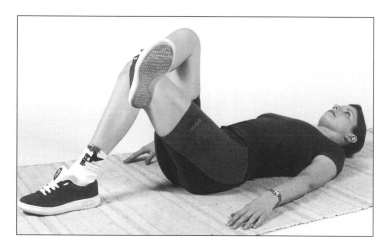

THE NEXT 2 EXERCISES ARE PERFORMED LYING ON YOUR FRONT.

BACKWARD LEG LIFTS X 5 EACH LEG
(FIGURE 42, BELOW)
This exercise is excellent for the hamstrings, buttock muscles and lower paraspinal muscles.

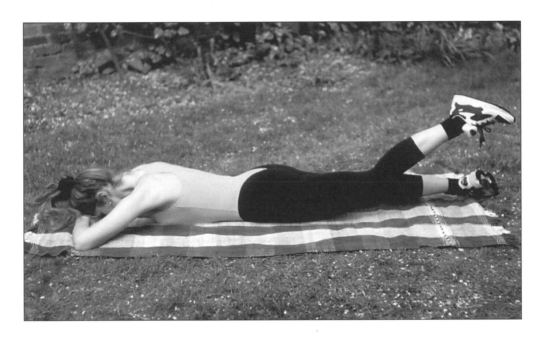

- Whilst lying on your front, place your hands folded in front of you, and rest your forehead on them.

- Keeping your hips as central and flat on the floor as possible, slowly lift one leg, held straight, up behind you. It is important that the strength of the movement comes from the buttock muscles and should not strain the lower back.

- Try not to arch the lower back during this exercise - it is primarily aimed at toning the backs of the legs and the buttocks.

Repeat the required number of times with the same leg, then move to the other.

HEAD AND SHOULDER LIFTS X 10
(FIGURE 43, BELOW)

This exercise is good for the upper paraspinal muscles, and also for the muscles of the upper arms, especially the triceps.

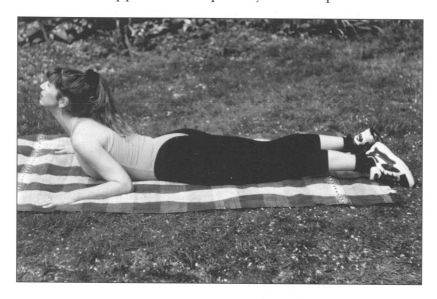

- Lie on your front with arms bent at the elbows, hands lying adjacent to shoulders (almost touching).

- Push down into the floor with your hands, and use this movement to lift your head and upper half of body about 10 inches off the floor.

- Throughout this movement, the forearm should be kept flat on the floor. Try to keep the hips flat on the floor.

Repeat.

SIDE LEG LIFTS X 10 EACH SIDE
(FIGURE 29, RIGHT, PAGE 107)

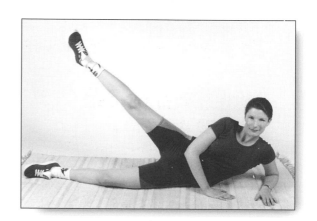

SECTION 3

Relax

Whilst still on the floor, roll again to lie on your back. Adopt the yoga relaxation position shown in Figure 16, Chapter 6.

ARM LIFTS X 6 EACH SIDE
(FIGURE 44, BELOW)

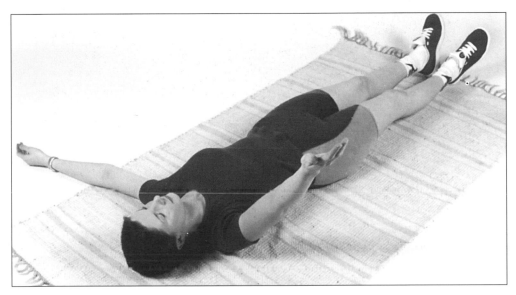

- Lie on your back with eyes closed and all muscles relaxed.

- Arms are stretched loosely out to the sides.

- Raise the right arm off the ground and slowly lower again.

Repeat then move to the other arm.

ANKLE CIRCLES X 10 EACH
SIDE AND DIRECTION
(FIGURE 32A, RIGHT, PAGE 112)

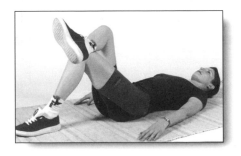

Now move to sit cross legged, with your back as upright as is comfortable.

CROSS-LEGGED FORWARD BENDS X 3
(FIGURE 45, BELOW)

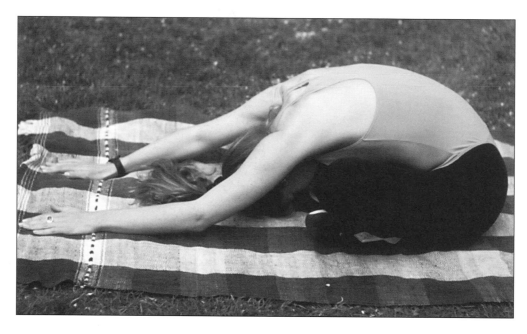

- Whilst sitting cross legged, slowly lean forwards with your back straight and arms stretched out in front of you.

- Breathe out as you lower your body down towards the floor, and in as you come up.

- Move to the standing position, with feet slightly apart, and with good posture.

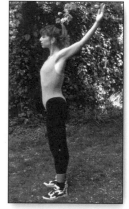

ARM CIRCLES X 3 BACKWARDS AND 3 FORWARDS
(FIGURE 33, RIGHT, PAGE 118)

SHAKE LEGS OUT
(FIGURE 46, BELOW)

This does not mean flinging your legs wildly at the hips and knees. This is a controlled movement with each leg in turn.

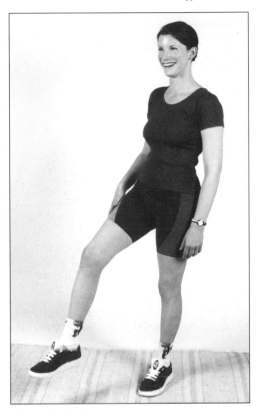

- Standing on one leg, supported if necessary with a hand placed on the back of a chair, gently bend the other leg at the hip.

- Slowly bend and straighten the leg several times at the knee.

Repeat with the other leg.

If you wish, you can continue to unwind and relax using the exercises shown in Chapter 5. Once you have mastered these exercises, you will be ready to move on to the more demanding ones shown in the next chapter.

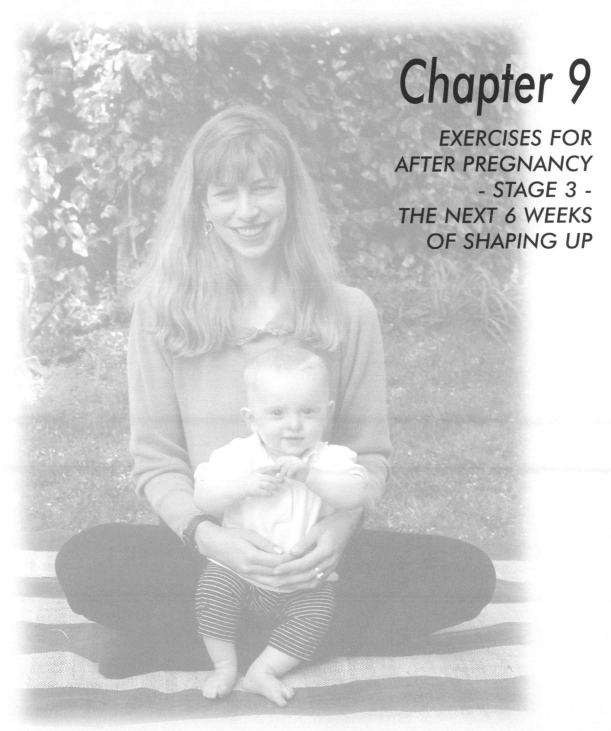

Chapter 9

EXERCISES FOR
AFTER PREGNANCY
- STAGE 3 -
THE NEXT 6 WEEKS
OF SHAPING UP

CHECKLIST

Warm Up

A: *Standing Exercises*

- Shoulder shrugs
- Chest hugs
- Elbow squeeze
- Hip presses
- Quarter waist turns
- High knee lifts

B: *Chair Exercises*

- Forward leg lifts
- Easy side leg lifts
- Waist twists
- Thigh rotations
- Controlled squats

C: *Dumb Bell Exercises*

- Shoulder girdle
- Alternating bicep curls
- Double tricep kick-backs
- Single arm extensions
- Double arm extensions
- Waist side-bends
- Forward lunges

D: Floor Exercises

- Bottom and adductor squeeze
- Knee waist turns
- Centre curl-up

    Stage 2
    Stage 3

- Diagonal curl-up

    Stage 2
    Stage 3

- Leg scissors
- Ankle circles
- Side leg lifts
- Head and shoulder lifts
- Backward leg lifts
- Buttock and pelvic squeeze

E: Relax

- Arm lifts
- Ankle circles
- Cross-legged forward bend
- Arm circles
- Shake legs out

By now, having completed and mastered the exercise routine shown in the previous chapter, many of your muscles will be gaining strength and should be on the way to becoming well-toned! The gap between the rectus muscles should have come together, and the discomfort in the perineum should have subsided. If the rectus muscles have not yet come together, continue to do the abdominal exercises shown on page 124 before moving on to the harder curl-ups and abdominal exercises shown here.

> **By the time you are ready to start the exercises in this section, any backache should have lessened. However, some ligaments in the spine may still not have recovered completely. All exercises should therefore continue (as always) to be performed carefully and without sudden movements to the spine or neck.**

Continue to do the pelvic floor exercises as often as you can. Contrast relaxation exercises (pp 83-84) can be performed in any position and are good for general toning of local muscle groups. In this chapter, the exercises shown in the routine in Chapter 8 will be added to, with the aim of working certain muscle groups harder. New exercises are also introduced which work the pectoral muscles and the muscles at the back of the arms (the triceps) and shoulders, in addition to further exercises for the hips and upper thighs.

In addition to the muscle strengthening and toning exercises shown here, you should now be ready to begin some form of aerobic exercise, to increase you cardiovascular fitness, and also to help you lose weight, if you need to. Walking and regular swimming are very effective and probably the most practical forms of aerobic exercise for this stage.

SECTION 1: *The Warm Up*

This is the same as that shown in Chapter 8.

SECTION 2 *Muscle Toning And Strengthening*
A: Standing exercises

SHOULDER SHRUGS X 10
(FIGURE 9, RIGHT, PAGE 76)

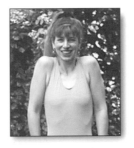

CHEST HUGS X 10
(FIGURE 36, RIGHT, PAGE 121)

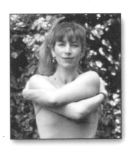

ELBOW SQUEEZE X 10
(FIGURE 47, RIGHT)

This exercise is excellent for the pectoral muscles in the chest.

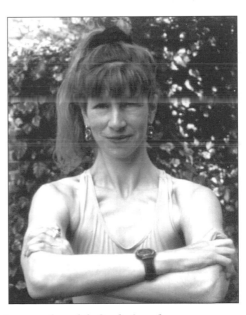

- Stand with your feet slightly apart.
- Check posture.
- Raise your arms directly out in front of you, parallel to the floor, palms facing downwards.
- Bend the arms at the elbows, bringing each hand to grasp the opposite arm, just above the elbow.
- Now push briskly with each hand against the opposite upper arm.

Count for 3 and release.

Repeat this movement rhythmically, and you should feel (and some women will also be able to see) the pectoral muscles appear and contract at the upper outer part of the chest wall above the breasts.

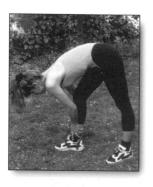

HIP PRESSES AND DIAGONAL TRUNK BENDS X 10 EACH SIDE
(FIGURE 37, LEFT, PAGE 122)

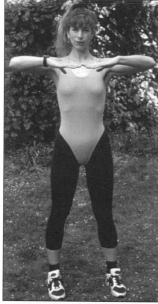

QUARTER WAIST TURNS X 10
(FIGURE 48, LEFT AND BELOW)

This exercise is excellent for the waist. It uses all the abdominal muscles, especially the obliques, the paraspinal muscles, and those of the arms and shoulder girdles.

- Stand with feet slightly apart.

- Bend your arms at the elbow, with finger tips almost meeting in front of you.

- Elbows should be held out at shoulder level. Keep your hips facing forwards throughout the exercise.

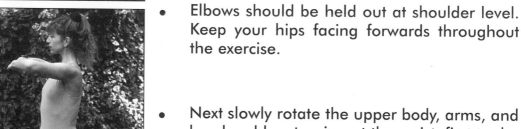

- Next slowly rotate the upper body, arms, and head en bloc, turning at the waist, first to the left (for the count of '1 and'), back to the centre (for the count of '2 and'), and then to the right ('3 and').

The movement should be slow and controlled. Take great care not to twist the spine forcefully.

HIGH KNEE LIFTS X 20 EACH SIDE
(FIGURES 49A AND 49B, BELOW)

This exercise is excellent for the abdominal muscles, the thighs, and also for the buttock muscles.

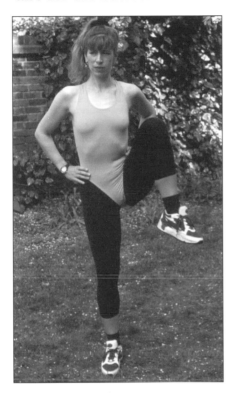 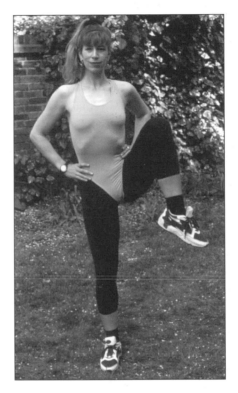

- Check posture.

- Stand with feet very slightly apart, and place your hands on your waist.

- Lift the left leg with the knee bent so that the knee comes as close as possible to touching the breast on that side.

- The toes of the foot should be pointed. This movement will undo the arch of the lower back, and will require a lot of support from the other leg. Hold on to a chair if you prefer, but take care not to lean in to it.

- Lower the leg back to the floor and repeat with the other leg.

B: Chair Exercises

For these exercises you will need a high-backed firm chair. In all cases where holding the chair with one hand is indicated, the chair should be used as a support and not a crutch.

FORWARD LEG LIFTS X 10 EACH SIDE
(FIGURE 50, BELOW)

This exercise is good for the abdominal muscles, the muscles at the front of the thigh (the quadriceps), the hip flexors, and the muscles of the buttocks.

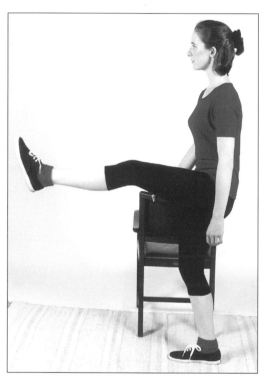

- Stand with one side of your body facing the chair.

- Make sure that the supporting knee is locked but not pushed back, and try not to lean your weight into the chair. Your back should be upright and the hips should be facing forwards.

- Hold the back of the chair with the hand nearest to it.

- Lift the leg furthest from the chair upwards and forwards, with the knee very slightly bent. The toes should not be pointed, but should be cocked upwards.

- The leg is then lowered so that the foot just touches the floor, but weight should not be transferred on to that foot.

- The raising and lowering is repeated with the same leg for the required number of times.

- The movements should be controlled and should not disintegrate into a swinging movement.

EASY SIDE LEG LIFTS X 10 EACH SIDE
(FIGURE 51, BELOW)
This exercise is good for the muscles on the outer aspect of the thighs, the buttocks and also the abdominal muscles.

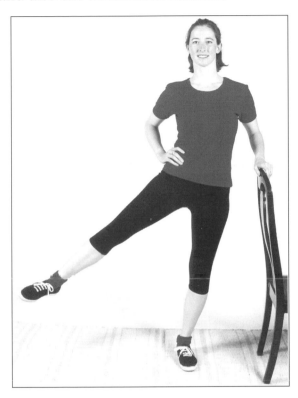

- Stand in the same starting position as in figure 50.

- With your weight on the leg nearest the chair, bend the other leg slightly at the knee. Take care not to lean into the chair.

- Lift the outer leg out to the side as far as it will go comfortably, with the knee straight. Make sure that your hips and shoulders are level and facing forwards.

- Lower the leg so that the foot just touches the floor.

- Repeat the up and down movements without transferring weight on to the outer foot in between each leg lift. The movements should be controlled and should not turn into a swing.

Repeat on the other side.

WAIST TWISTS X 10 EACH SIDE
(FIGURES 52A AND 52B, BELOW)

This exercise helps to firm the waist and also uses the muscles running along the spine. It should be done slowly and carefully so as not to twist the spine forcibly.

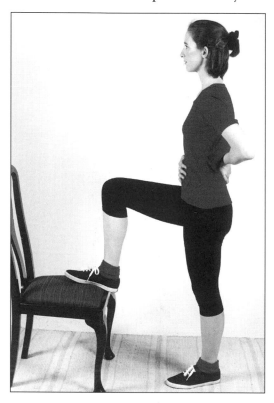 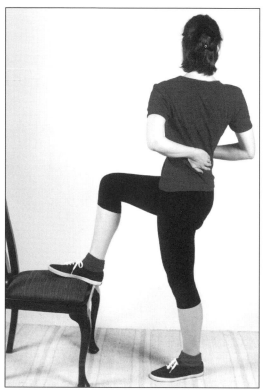

- Stand facing the seat of the chair and place one foot on the seat.

- Place the palm of your right hand on your tummy, and place the palm of your left hand on the lower back.

- Gently turn the upper part of your body towards the right (do not swing or bounce), making sure that your shoulders remain level, and trying to keep your hips facing the chair. Your head and neck should move with your shoulders.

- Return slowly to centre and repeat for the required number on that side. Then change hands.

Reverse leg positions, and repeat to the other side.

THIGH ROTATIONS X 10 EACH LEG
(FIGURES 53A AND 53B, BELOW)
This exercise uses the thigh muscles including those that run along the inside of the leg (the abductors).

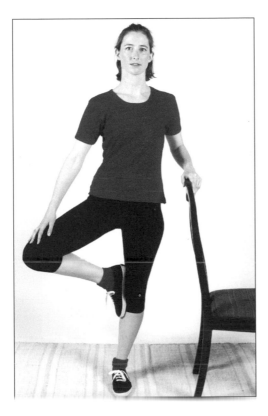 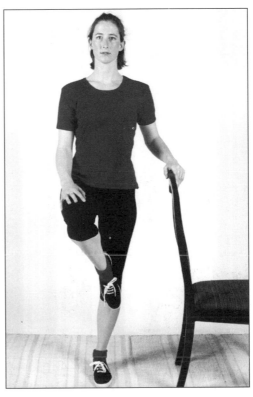

- Stand holding the back of the chair as for the forward leg lifts (figure 50).

- Bend the leg furthest from the chair at the knee and place the sole of the foot of that leg on the inside of the knee.

- Slowly rotate the bent knee through a 90° angle forwards and then out to the side again and backwards as far as is comfortable.

- This movement should involve active contraction of all muscles at the upper part of the thigh and pelvic area.

Repeat the required number of times, and then change over to the other side.

CONTROLLED SQUATS X 10

(FIGURE 54, BELOW)

This exercise is excellent for the thigh muscles, but is also good for the muscles of the calves and back.

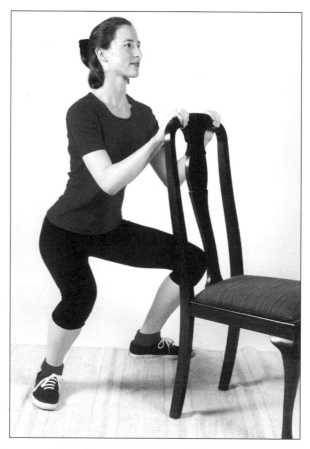

- Stand with your feet just over shoulder width apart, facing the back of the chair, with both hands resting on it.

- With your back straight, lower yourself down by bending at the knees, until the thighs are roughly parallel with the floor (i.e. your thigh and calves are at right angles). Your knees should be directly above the ankles and feet should remain flat on the floor.

- Hold for a count of '1 and' and slowly come up again.

C: Dumb Bell Exercises

The muscles in the arms and shoulders in women can look beautiful if they are properly toned. It is relatively easy to get them into that shape using these exercises. These exercises use 3 pound dumb bells, and are not aimed at building muscle. However, they will definitely help to make your muscles in the arms and upper part of the body better defined and 'strong' looking. There is nothing to be gained by doing dumb bell exercises fast (other than strained muscles!), so ensure that all are done slowly and with control.

The following group of 5 exercises strengthen the upper arm and chest. The exercises shown in figures 57-59 strengthen and tone the triceps muscle at the back of the upper arm. This muscle has a tendency to become flabby with age and the upper arm is also an area where fat tends to collect during pregnancy.

- Alternating bicep curls

- Double tricep kick-backs

- Single arm extensions

- Double arm extensions

- Waist side-bends

SHOULDER GIRDLE X 10

(FIGURES 55A AND 55B, BELOW)

This exercise uses the muscles of the shoulder girdle and upper arm.

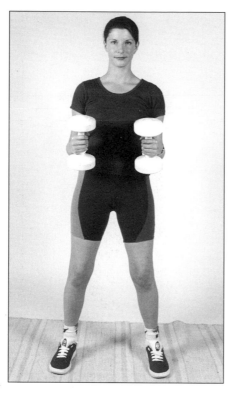 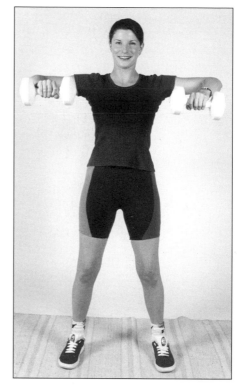

- Stand with your feet about shoulder width apart.

- Hold one weight in each hand, with arms bent at the elbows at 90 degrees.

- Start with the elbows tucked into the waist. Check posture and bend knees very slightly.

- Raise your elbows out to the side, keeping them bent at the same angle throughout, to just above shoulder height.

- Do the upward movement to a count of '1 and', hold in the 'up' position for a count of '2 and', and then return to the lower position to a count of '3 and', resting in between each cycle for a count of '4 and'.

Repeat.

> **If you find this exercise too tiring to start with, try reducing the number of cycles or use smaller weights, and do only one arm at a time, whilst the other hand is resting on the back of a chair.**

ALTERNATING BICEPS CURLS

(FIGURES 56A AND 56B, BELOW)

As its name suggests, this exercise uses the biceps muscle in the upper arm.

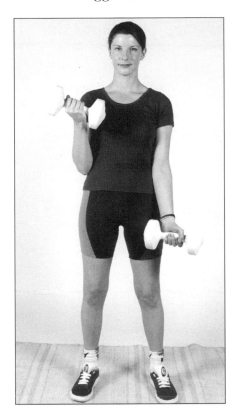 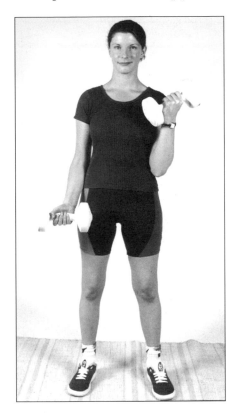

- Stand with your feet just about shoulder width apart, knees slightly bent.

- Check posture. Hold one weight in each hand with the palms of your hands facing forwards, and keep your elbows tucked into your waist throughout the exercise.

- Raise one weight up as far as you can by bending the arm at the elbow, so that your hand comes up towards your shoulder.

- Lower that arm, and as you do so, bring the opposite weight up using the other hand, in the same way. Continue the cycles in a steady smooth stream.

Note: The downward movement is as important as the upward movement (resisting the effect of gravity) and should be done slowly.

DOUBLE TRICEP KICK-BACKS
(FIGURES 57A AND 57B, BELOW)

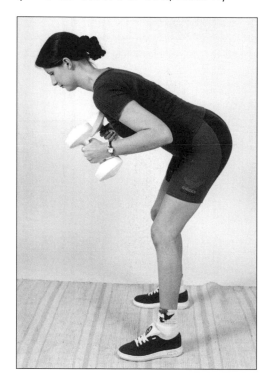 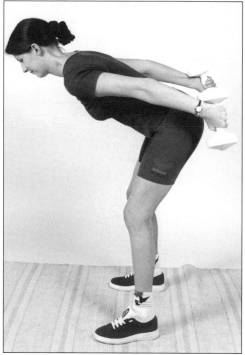

- Stand with feet pointing forwards, about shoulder width apart.

- Bend knees slightly, and bend your upper body forwards at the hips so that your shoulders are above your feet.

- Hold a dumb bell in each hand, elbows slightly bent, with elbows pointing out behind you. Once your back is braced steadily on your legs, lift the dumb bells back and upwards by straightening the arms out behind you as far as they will comfortably go, to a count of '1 and'.

- The palms of the hands should be facing the floor at the end of this movement. Hold in that 'up' position for a count of '2 and' and then return slowly to the count of '3 and' to the starting position, where you rest for a count of '4 and'.

Repeat.

SINGLE ARM EXTENSIONS
(FIGURES 58A AND 58B, BELOW)

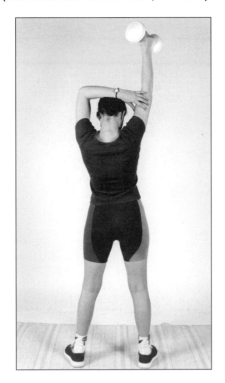 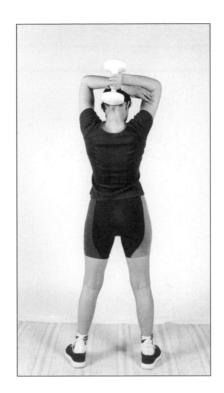

- Stand with feet shoulder width apart, knees bent slightly.

- Holding a weight in one hand, lift the arm so that the dumb bell is directly above your head.

- Bring the other arm up to the same position and bend it at the elbow, clasping the area just above the elbow of the arm holding the weight. This will act as a support.

- The supporting arm should be gently resting on the forehead.

- Slowly bend the arm holding the dumb bell at the elbow, so that the forearm rests on the opposite supporting hand.

- Raise the weight slowly and repeat. The dumb bell should lower behind your head, and as it does so, take care not to hit yourself with it!

Reverse arm position and repeat with the other side.

DOUBLE ARM EXTENSIONS
(FIGURES 59A AND 59B, BELOW)

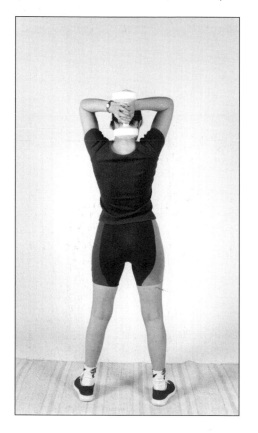 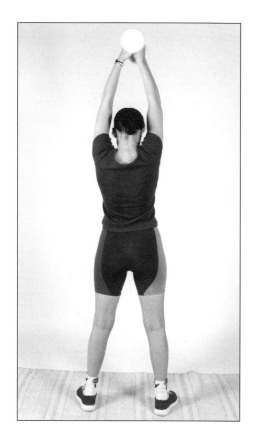

- Stand as in figure 58.

- Hold a single dumb bell with both hands, placing it behind your head. Try not to bend your head forwards.

- Slowly raise the weight directly upwards (and not forwards in an arc) with both hands as far as you can above your head, taking care not to lock the elbows in a straight position.

Return to starting position and repeat.

WAIST SIDE-BENDS

(FIGURES 60A AND 60B, BELOW)

This exercise uses all the muscles on one side of the abdomen, together with the muscles running the length of the spine. It is excellent for the waist.

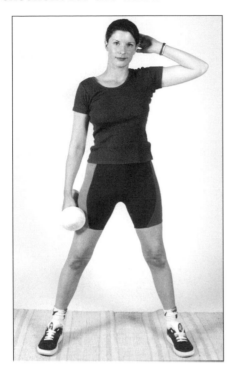 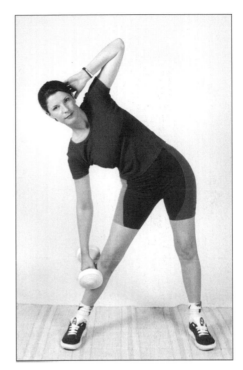

- Stand with feet shoulder width apart.

- Hold a dumb bell in one hand, with the arm hanging down by your side, palm facing inwards.

- Raise the hand not holding the weight and place it on the side of your head.

- Reach down sideways (on the side of the dumb bell) so that the weight is level with your knee, whilst keeping the weight close to the side of the leg.

- Try to keep your back parallel with the plane of your legs, and make sure you do not lean forwards.

- Return to the starting position and repeat.

Change sides and repeat.

FORWARD LUNGES
(FIGURES 61A AND 61B, BELOW)

These exercises should only be attempted when your back has totally recovered and is already strengthened by completion of the foregoing exercises. The exercises are excellent for the back muscles, the thigh and buttock, as well as toning the abdomen.

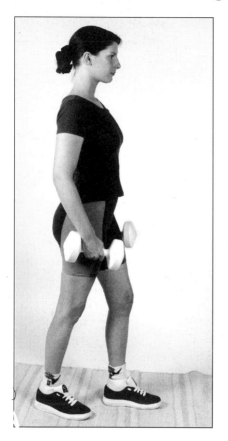
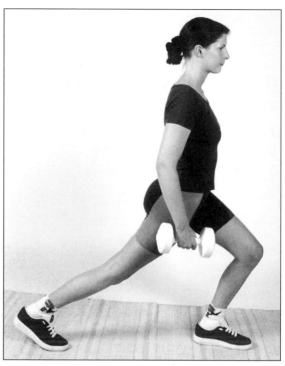

- Stand with your back straight, arms by your sides, holding a weight in each hand, and feet together.

- Take a step forward with one leg, bend at the knee, taking care not to bend the knee more than 90 degrees. Your back and neck should be straight.

- Stand straight again by pushing up off the forward bent leg.

Repeat with the opposite leg.

D: *Floor Exercises*

Lying on your back

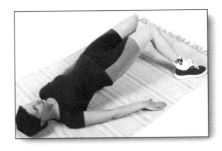

BOTTOM AND ADDUCTOR SQUEEZE X 10
(FIGURE 40, RIGHT, PAGE 126)

KNEE-WAIST TURNS X 20 EACH SIDE
(FIGURE 62, BELOW)

This exercise is excellent for the thighs, both inner and outer aspects, but especially for the outer parts at the tops of the thighs which have a tendency to become flabby; the exercise is also excellent for the waist.

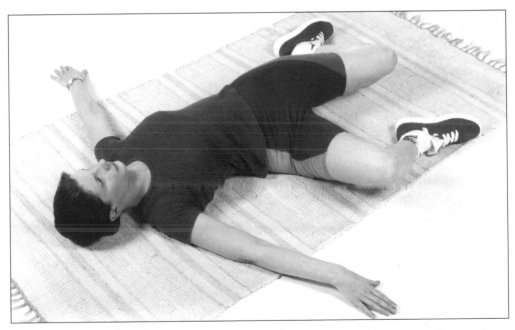

- Lie on your back with your arms stretched out to the sides, palms flat on the ground. Your legs should be bent at the knees, with your feet placed flat on the floor, and tucked to about 8 inches away from each cheek of your bottom.

- The legs and hips should feel comfortable.

cont'd...

- The sequence of movements involves rotating the right thigh outwards so that it comes close to lying on the floor on its outer surface.

- At the same time, the left leg is rotated inwards so that the knee comes close to touching the floor directly in front of where you are lying.

- The movements are then reversed (as shown below) so that the right knee is brought forwards to touch the floor, and the left thigh is rotated outwards to lie on its outer aspect on the floor.

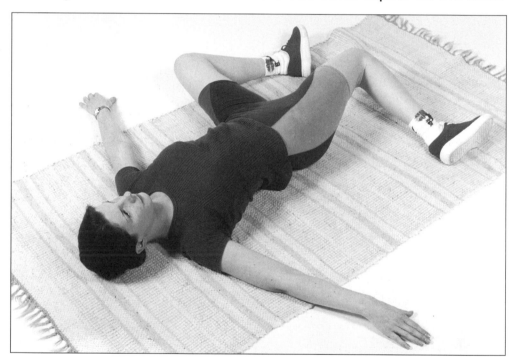

- These movements should be repeated rhythmically, but in a controlled manner, taking care not to twist the lower spine. The hips should roll very slightly throughout the movements of the legs.

Next come the curl-ups

I suggest you begin these exercises with the Stage 2 exercises only. Once these have been mastered, you can move on to Stage 3. These exercises are excellent for restoring the waist line and strengthening the abdomen; a strong abdomen also aids posture.

CENTRE CURL-UPS, STAGE 2, X 5 EACH SIDE
(FIGURE 63, BELOW)

The basic position is the same as Stage 1 centre curl-ups shown in figure 38, page 124.

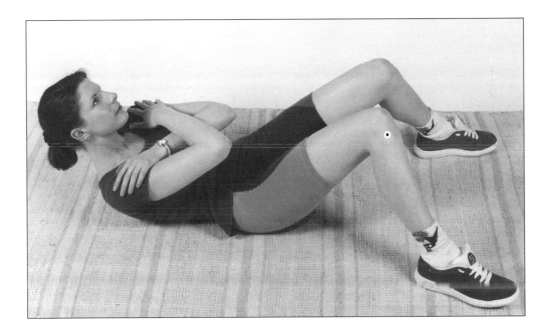

- However, now your arms are crossed over your chest, and each hand grips the opposite shoulder; alternatively it can grip the side of the waist.

- As you breathe out, lift your head and shoulders up off the floor attempting to look at your knees.

- Hold for a count of '3 and' then return slowly to the flat position (do not drop back suddenly), breathing in as you do so.

Repeat as required.

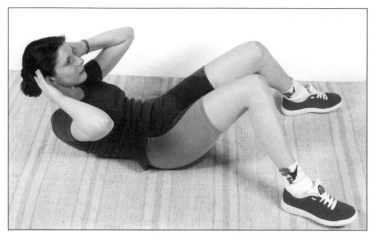

CENTRE CURL-UPS, STAGE 3, X 5 EACH SIDE
(FIGURE 64, LEFT)

This is exactly as for Stage 2 except that now the palms of the hands are placed gently over your ears, taking great care not to pull on your neck.

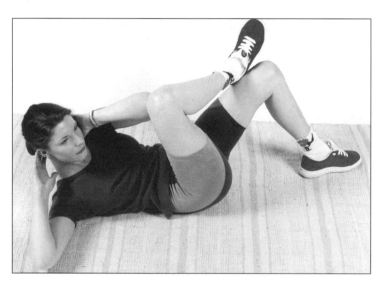

DIAGONAL CURL-UPS, STAGE 2, X 5 EACH SIDE
(FIGURE 65, LEFT)

- Lie on your back with knees bent and feet flat on the floor.
- Place each hand gently over one ear.
- Next rest the right ankle just above the left knee.
- Do a diagonal curl-up by lifting up your head and left shoulder, and attempt to touch the right knee with the left elbow.
- Return slowly to the starting position, and repeat on the same side the required number of times.

Then reverse leg positions and repeat with the other side.

DIAGONAL CURL-UPS, STAGE 3 X 5 EACH SIDE
(FIGURE 66, BELOW)

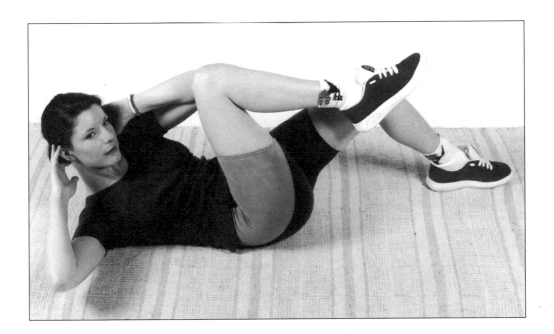

- Lie on your back with knees bent and feet flat on the floor, hands placed gently over your ears.

- Do a diagonal curl-up as in figure 65 (opposite), except this time the knee is lifted up towards the opposite elbow in an attempt to meet it.

This is repeated on the same side before changing to the opposite side.

LEG SCISSORS X 10
(FIGURES 67A AND 67B, BELOW)

This exercise strengthens the abdominal muscles and many of the thigh muscles.

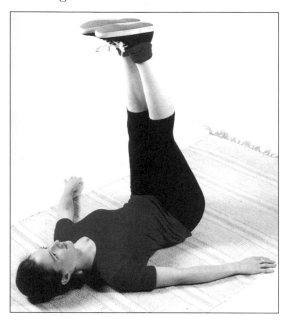 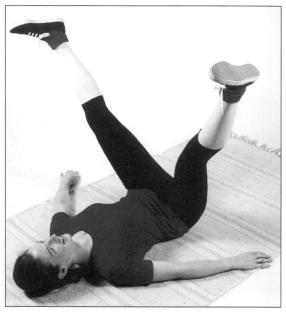

- Lie on your back with your arms stretched out to the sides, with palms of hands flat on the floor.

- Bend your legs at the knees and lift your feet off the floor.

- Straighten out at the knees as far as comfortable. It is important that your feet are above your hips.

- Slowly part your feet bringing them out to the sides so that the feet are level with the hands.

- Slowly bring the legs together in the midline so that the feet touch.

Repeat as required.

ANKLE CIRCLES X 10 EACH ANKLE AND EACH DIRECTION
(FIGURE 32, BELOW, PAGE 112)

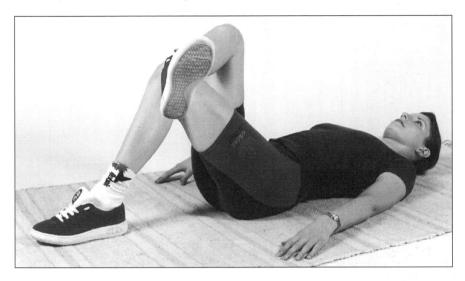

NOW TURN TO LIE ON YOUR SIDE.

SIDE LEG LIFTS - ABDUCTORS X 5 EACH SIDE
(FIGURE 29, BELOW, PAGE 107)

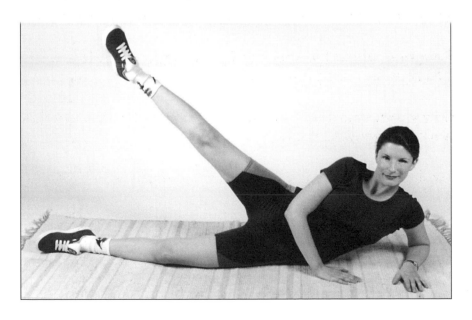

SIDE LEG LIFTS - ABDUCTORS X 5 EACH SIDE
(FIGURES 68A AND 68B, BELOW)

This exercise is excellent for the muscles running along the inner aspects of the thighs - the adductor muscles.

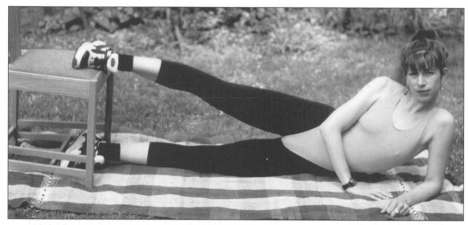

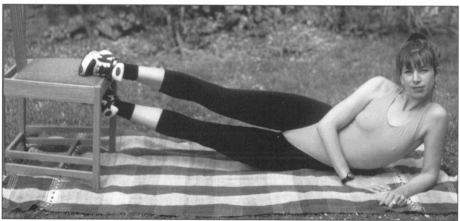

- Position yourself as in figure 29, page 107.

- Rest your upper-most foot on the seat of the chair.

- Slowly lift the lower foot up towards the upper foot (i.e. the under part of the chair) as far as you can, but keeping your body perpendicular with the ground.

- Slowly lower the foot to the ground and repeat. Then change over to the other side.

NOW LIE ON YOUR FRONT.

HEAD AND SHOULDER LIFTS X 10
(FIGURE 43, BELOW, PAGE 130)

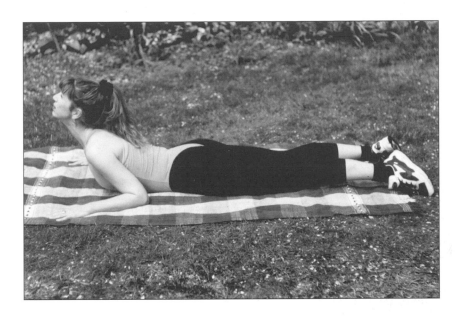

BACKWARD LEG LIFTS X 5 EACH SIDE
(FIGURE 42, BELOW, PAGE 129)

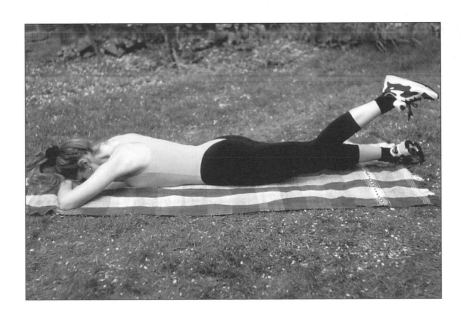

BUTTOCK AND PELVIC SQUEEZE X 5
(FIGURE 69, BELOW)

This exercise tones the bottom and all of the pelvic floor muscles.

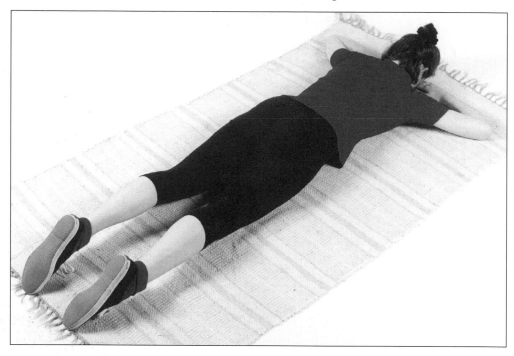

- Lie on your front, and gently rest your chin on your hands, which should be resting palm down on the floor in front of your face.

- Squeeze your buttock muscles and the pelvic floor firmly together at the same time as curling your pubic bone down towards the floor.

- You should feel your abdominal muscles contracting as you do this, and a gap should appear between your abdomen and the floor as your muscles contract.

Release and repeat.

Relax

Whilst still lying on the floor, roll on to your back and adopt the relaxed yoga position showed in figure 16, pages 84-85.

ARM LIFTS X 3 EACH SIDE
(FIGURE 44, RIGHT, PAGE 131)

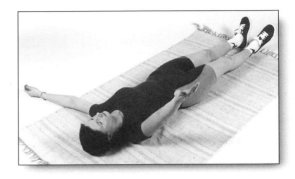

ANKLE CIRCLES X 3 EACH SIDE AND EACH DIRECTION
(FIGURE 41, RIGHT, PAGE 128)

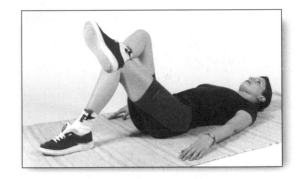

MOVE TO THE SITTING POSITION WITH CROSSED LEGS.

CROSS LEGGED FORWARD BEND X 3
(FIGURE 45, RIGHT, PAGE 132)

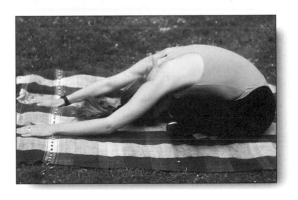

STAND UP AND CHECK POSTURE

ARM CIRCLES X 3 BACKWARDS EACH SIDE
(FIGURE 33, BELOW, PAGE 118)

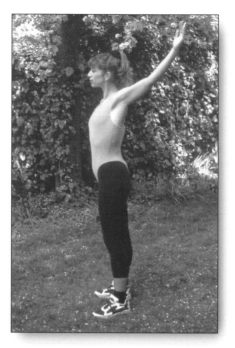

SHAKE LEGS OUT
(FIGURE 46, BELOW, PAGE 133)

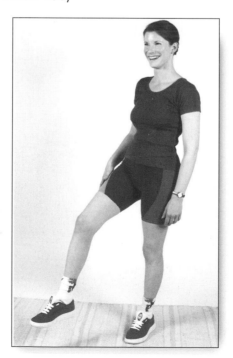

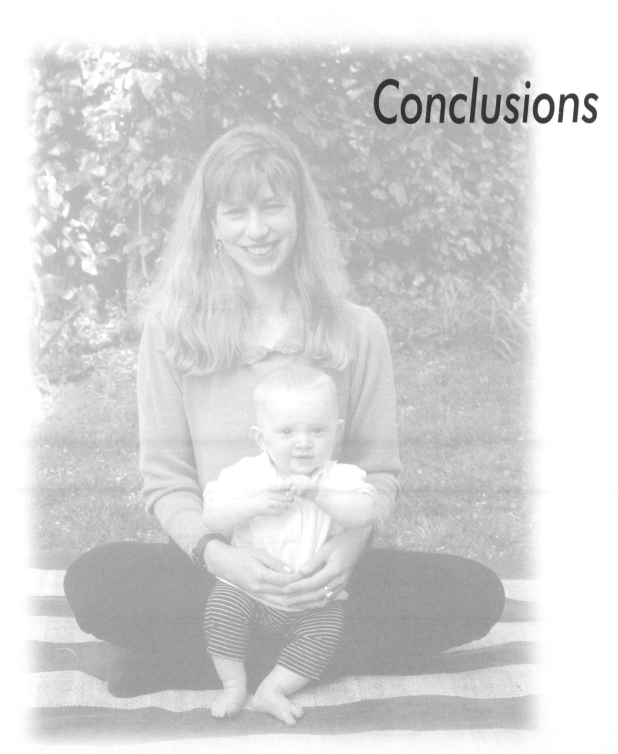

Conclusions

CONCLUSIONS

All women are different, and some regain their pre-pregnancy shape more readily and more completely than others. Some women also seem to have to try more than others.

However 'bad' you may feel you are at exercises, I am certain that if you have persevered with these exercises, and done them regularly, then the shape of your body, its strength and tone, will have improved markedly. Once you have mastered the exercise routines shown in this chapter, and are in the position where you can perform the exercises with ease and without referring to the book, you will have reached an excellent level of muscle strengthening and toning.

These exercises are designed to be continued for as long as you wish after delivery of your baby. They are worth re-starting even when you are well past delivery, if you should lose your newly sculpted form!

Whenever the regimes are started, remember to begin from the first stages shown in Chapter 7, and to build up. Practice the posture, breathing and relaxation exercises whenever you can.

The weeks and months following the birth of your baby can be one of the happiest and fulfiling periods of a mother's life. It is important that during this period you feel as content with yourself as you can, and this includes feeling healthy and feeling that you look good!

There is something particularly attractive about a woman with a young baby who also looks well toned and fit. Regular physical activity of the moderate sort described in this book will help you to achieve that goal. If you are lucky enough to have a friend who has also had a baby recently (or a friend who just wants to tone up) try and entice them to do the exercises with you on a regular basis.

Whatever else, this book should get you into shape effectively and painlessly. I hope you will enjoy using it.

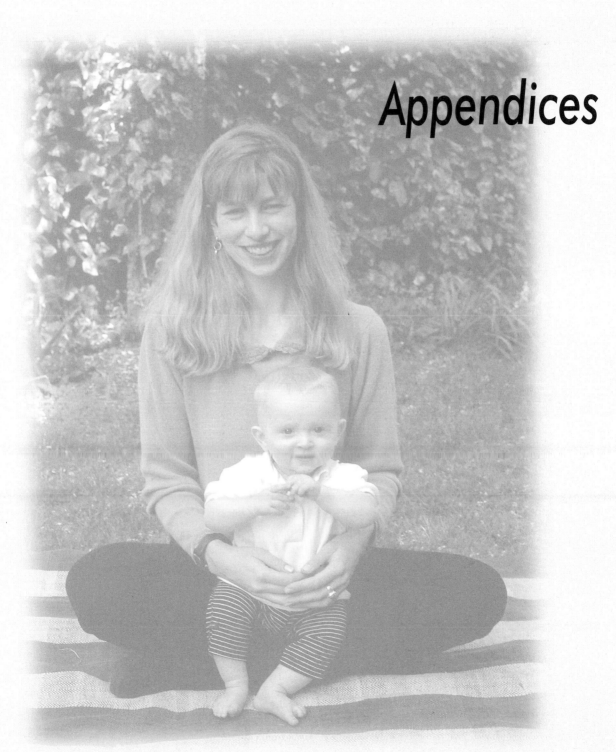

Appendices

APPENDIX I

Hormonal Changes During And After Pregnancy

It is the hormonal changes that are largely responsible for the changes that occur to the mother's body during reproduction. It is important therefore to understand these changes, but if there is anything that you are unsure about, then consult your GP. The following additional information on some of the hormones should further your understanding of both physical and psychological changes.

OESTROGENS

In addition to the effects on breasts and uterus (page 16), oestrogens are also responsible for the distribution of fat seen in women, and exemplified in the pregnant and breast-feeding woman: fat tends to be deposited especially in the breasts, upper arms, upper thighs, hips and bottom. A layer of fat which tends to accumulate over the hips during pregnancy is thought to be important in providing fat stores which can be drawn on to provide energy during breast feeding. Oestrogens are also probably responsible for the comparatively high ratio of head-to-body hair that is found in women. Oestrogens also have more general effects such as improving the strength of bones and preventing osteoporosis and promoting blood clotting.

Although oestrogens are mainly produced by the ovaries, some forms are produced in other parts of the body, in particular fat and muscle. It is for this reason that the amount of body fat (as a percentage of total body weight) is important in fertility: too little fat, or too much, can both have harmful effects on the reproductive capacity of a woman.

HUMAN CHORIONIC GONADOTROPHIN

Human chorionic gonadotrophin (HCG) is produced from very early stages in pregnancy by the placenta, and measurement of its level in the blood or urine is the basis of the most sensitive pregnancy tests. The levels increase steadily up to week 20 of pregnancy, at which time they level off.

HUMAN PLACENTAL LACTOGEN

Human placental lactogen (HPL) is another hormone which is specific to pregnancy. It is produced by the placenta, and its levels in the mother's blood increase progressively towards the end of pregnancy.

OXYTOCIN

When the baby sucks on the breast, a message is sent from the breast to the pituitary gland in the brain, which triggers the release of oxytocin. Oxytocin travels in the blood back to the breast where it stimulates the muscle cells around the glands to contract, and so eject the milk. This effect of suckling also means that oxytocin released into the blood travels to other parts of the body, including the uterus. Here it will cause increased contractions of the uterus (so-called 'after-pains') which, whilst uncomfortable, are an effective way of encouraging the shrinkage of the uterus that normally occurs after delivery.

PROLACTIN

High levels of prolactin are found after pregnancy when milk production is being established, and levels remain high if breast-feeding continues. Prolactin inhibits the production of eggs by the ovaries, and so is partly responsible for the 'contraceptive' effect of breast-feeding (although this method of contraception should not be relied on alone).

RELAXIN

This hormone is found in the ovary during pregnancy and may play an important role during delivery, although its exact role in humans is uncertain. One view is that, together with oestrogen and progesterone, relaxing causes relaxation of the ligaments of the pelvic bones and a softening of the cervix, which may help with the passage of the baby through the birth canal. During pregnancy, relaxing may also be responsible for the relaxation of other ligaments, including those of the spine. These effects may account for the poor posture that often occurs during pregnancy.

OTHER HORMONES

In particular, levels of thyroid hormones increase, as do those produced by the adrenal glands. Higher levels of adrenal corticosteroids are produced during pregnancy and these may contribute to the tendency to form stretch marks over the abdomen and elsewhere. Higher levels of insulin are also produced during pregnancy.

APPENDIX II

Nutrition And Diet During Pregnancy

Concern with weight and physical appearance is probably at its greatest after birth. Nutrition and diet play a very important part in losing any excess weight.

> **The food allowances recommended in this book are based on the Recommended Dietary Allowances (RDAs) of the Food and Nutrition Board of the National Academy of Sciences. The RDAs vary according to sex, age and reproductive state: here the values relate only to women of reproductive age.**

Depending on body size and level of physical activity, the average number of calories required for a medium-framed non-pregnant woman ranges from 2000-2400 calories per day. Calorie requirements during pregnancy increase because the mother needs energy for herself as well as for the growing fetus. The energy requirements do not, however, increase by as much as we might think! During the first three months of pregnancy, energy requirements do not significantly increase above those of pre-pregnancy, but in the second and third trimesters, it is recommended that the daily calorie intake should increase by 300. During breast-feeding, the calorie requirements increase by a further 200 per day.

APPENDIX III

Mineral And Trace Element Requirements During Pregnancy

Most mineral and trace elements are readily available in a normal balanced diet. The following four are those most likely to become deficient and so RDA's are given.

IRON

During pregnancy, women should ensure that their diet contains approximately 30mg/ day of iron, but up to 60mg/ day is needed if they are iron-deficient at the onset of pregnancy. In the non-pregnant and no-breast-feeding state, the RDA for iron is 15mg. Balanced diets will provide adequate amounts of iron, and supplements are not usually required. Vitamin C greatly increases the amount of iron absorbed from certain types of foods eaten at the same meal.

CALCIUM

Vitamin D is formed in the skin by the effect of sunlight, and this process can be reduced in dark skinned people, especially when the level of sunlight is low (as in the UK in winter). During pregnancy, when demands are high, Vitamin D deficiency, and consequently low calcium levels in the body, can occur quite easily. It is therefore important to ensure that sufficient amounts of food are eaten which contain calcium and are fortified with Vitamin D.

ZINC

During pregnancy, about 5% of the whole body content of zinc is retained in the baby and in the maternal tissues of pregnancy, so the zinc requirements increase and it is advisable for pregnant women to consume 15mg of zinc per day. This amount is easily achieved in a balanced diet, although vegetarians are at risk of dietary deficiency. Zinc supplementation is not routinely recommended during pregnancy, but it should be taken if iron supplements at a dose of 60mg per day are being consumed.

APPENDIX IV

Effects Of Diet Restriction And Weight Gain During Pregnancy

Dieting during pregnancy is not advisable. The following information will further your understanding of recommended weight gain.

Although the fetus tends to draw on maternal stores when the diet of the mother is restricted, the extent to which this occurs is uncertain. Mild dietary restriction initially occurs at the expense of the mother's weight. Once the mother's weight has fallen below a critical threshold, or once diet is severely restricted to 'starvation' levels (e.g. below 800 calories per day), fetal health is seriously at risk. At that point, diet restriction during pregnancy seems to affect the mother's weight proportionately less than the developing baby. Inadequate diet seems to be most harmful to the baby during the third trimester, when fetal growth should be most rapid.